In honor of the unwavering dedication and boundless love of my life,

Dr. Sheena Kuriakose,

and our fitness enthusiast son, **Jovit J Sebastian**,

whose passion for health and wellness inspires every page of this book

YOUR BODY TELLS YOUR LIFE STORY

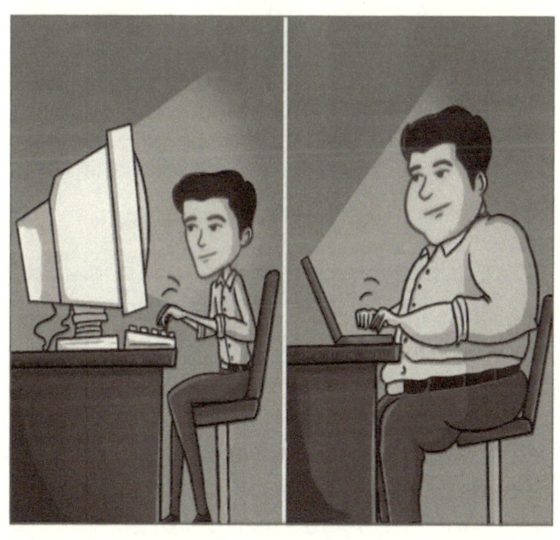

DR. JINO SEBASTIAN

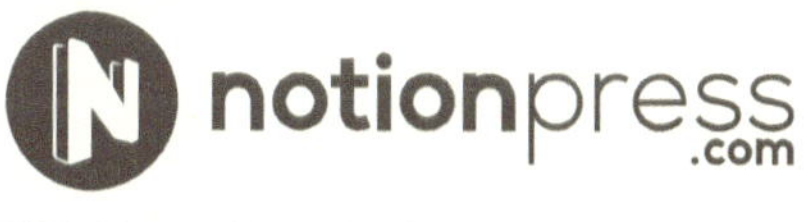

INDIA · SINGAPORE · MALAYSIA

ISBN 979-8-89133-830-2

Contents

Introduction

Our society is facing some serious problems. Not many of us are getting enough exercise, and this is causing more and more people to become overweight. This can lead to heart problems and diabetes, which are becoming more common. The air we breathe is also not very clean, and it's hurting our lungs. More and more children are not getting enough food to eat, and this is a big concern. In schools, kids have less space to play and are spending more time in front of screens, which is making these problems even worse. Anxiety and sadness are also becoming more common in our society. We need to work together to find solutions to these issues and make our lives healthier and happier.

The only remedy for the above problem is regular exercise and proper nutrition. Regularity in exercise must be like brushing the teeth and attending the natures call. We regularly take food in a certain interval but we are very lazy towards exercise. "If there is a will there is way" is quite applicable in the case of exercise, exercise can be done with minimum space, that can be done in our bed room or office room. Even five minutes of exercise can elevate our mood in a great manner. We are good spectators of sport but reluctant to participate.

Nutrition is as important as exercise for human health. Jack Lalanne said it well: "Exercise is the king and nutrition is the queen. Put them together you've got a kingdom". We need to know the nutritional needs of our body and the nutritional value of food items to maintain a balanced diet. If the fuel is not suitable for the machine, it will not work well and will break down after some time. We will get sick and inefficient if we keep disrespecting our body. Proper exercise and nutrition can release happy hormones like endorphin, serotonin and oxytocin.

The aim of education is to develop the student holistically. However, the current education system focuses only on intellectual development. Other aspects like physical, mental, social, emotional developments are ignored. Today's generation is dependent on tuition and their talents are only judged by their academic grade.

Welcome to my comprehensive guide to physical fitness and nutrition! This book is designed to provide you with the knowledge and tools you need to achieve optimal health and wellness through a combination of exercise and healthy eating.

Physical fitness and nutrition are two sides of the same coin. Exercise is essential for building strength, improving cardiovascular health, and maintaining a healthy weight. Proper nutrition, on the other hand, is essential for providing your body with the nutrients it needs to fuel your workouts and support overall health and well-being. I hope that you find it informative, inspiring, and above all, useful in helping you achieve your fitness and nutrition goals.

Indeed, it's important to remember that the journey towards fitness is more like an endurance event than a sprint. Just as drops of water gradually form an ocean, the accumulation of consistent fitness activities will ultimately lead you to a state of improved fitness and well-being.

1

Physical Fitness

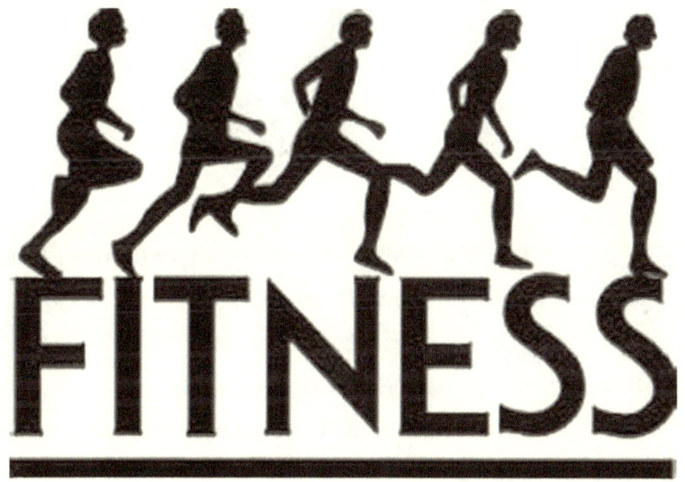

"The doctors of the future will give no medicine, but will interest his patients in the care of human frame, in diet, and in the cause and prevention of disease"

–Thomas Edison (American Inventor & businessmen)

Although we study a wide range of subjects, we often neglect to learn about the most complex machine of all: the human body. Unlike with electronic equipment, where we tend to read the user's manual immediately after purchase, we tend to use our bodies without understanding their basic functions. This lack of knowledge can lead to hypokinetic diseases, anxiety, and stress. It's important to recognize that wealth is meaningless without good health, much like a good hat is of no use if your head has been chopped off. Therefore, it's essential to prioritize learning about our own bodies and how they function.

The chance to burn the calories by physical activity is reducing day by day. We have cars for long journey, two wheelers for short journey, muti storied buildings with lifts and escalators, pavements in the cities are occupied either by hawkers or parking. Obesity is a multifaceted issue that goes beyond what is visible on the surface. In order to prevent obesity, we need to create environments that encourage physical activity. This can include playgrounds in schools, roads with designated bike lanes, and neighborhoods with parks. While having a bit of extra weight may be advantageous in certain situations, such as during a major illness or in old age, it is important to maintain a healthy weight throughout life.

With each passing day, it seems that people are becoming less active and increasingly sedentary. Some have even started parking their cars inside their homes, contributing to a decrease in daily steps taken. Unfortunately, this trend, coupled with a diet heavy in junk and fried foods, is causing people's bodies to become flabby and unhealthy. To make matters worse, some parents mistakenly believe that their children's obesity is a sign of wealth.

Namboodiri is a skilled craftsman who was sculpting an idol of Lord Krishna out of a piece of wood. When someone inquired about the idol, he replied that he had carefully removed everything except for the essence of Lord Krishna from the wood. Similarly, in order to achieve a healthy body, we must eliminate unwanted fat through a balanced diet and regular physical activity. By doing so, we can maintain our pride and confidence within ourselves.

Just like a watch that requires many parts to work together in synchronization to keep accurate time, the organs in our body, such as the heart, lungs, brain, and liver, need to function in a coordinated manner. If there is any interference, such as dust, water, or low battery, the watch won't work properly, and similarly, if there is a malfunction in any of our organs, it can affect our overall health and wellbeing.

Modern conveniences, such as microwave ovens, computers, cars, power tools, washers and dryers, have made our lives easier. However, parents are now struggling to get their kids out of the house to play, which is the opposite of what used to be in the past. Hypokinetic diseases, like obesity and diabetes, are starting to affect children at an early age. This is likely due to the fact that town life and nuclear families have led to a decrease in physical activity, with many children spending most of their time in social media and playing video games.

It's important for children to engage in play, just as outdoor plants are able to thrive in different climates. However, indoor plants are not always as successful. In the same way, playing outdoors can boost a child's immunity and resistance to disease.

Just as building a house requires a team of skilled professionals, such as carpenters, masons, and plumbers, working together in harmony, our bodies also require various systems, including the circulatory, respiratory, and digestive systems, to work in tandem in order to maintain good health and achieve optimal functionality. Without this coordinated effort, our bodies may struggle to operate efficiently and effectively. In the case of a violin, the strings need to work together to produce beautiful sounds. Each component has an important role to play, and the combination of both creates something greater than the sum of its parts.

The human body is designed to function like a well-oiled machine, with joints meant to move in a specific way. This is similar to a machine that was developed to operate in a particular manner, and cannot be manipulated outside of its intended design. However, our ancestors engaged in a variety of functional movements, including climbing, running, twisting, bending, and more. Nowadays, we may not engage in as many of these movements, which can impact our overall physical health and wellbeing.

If we consider the pumping motor of the human body, the heart begins to beat at 72 beats per minute, starting from 22 days in the mother's womb. By the time a person reaches the age of 70, their heart will have beaten approximately 260 crores times without a single day off or holiday. During each beat, the heart works for approximately 0.32 seconds and then takes a rest for around 0.48 seconds. It's truly amazing to think about the nonstop work our hearts do to keep us alive.

The heart is not just a physical organ that pumps blood throughout our body; it is also an emotional center that plays a vital role in our overall health and well-being. Emotions such as love, compassion, and acceptance have a direct impact on our heart health.

When we experience positive emotions, such as love and compassion, our heart rate and blood pressure tend to decrease, which can have a positive effect on our overall cardiovascular health. Conversely, negative emotions such as grief and stress can increase our heart rate and blood pressure, which can put a strain on our heart over time.

In addition to its emotional role, the heart is also one of the most selfless organs in our body. It continually pumps oxygen-rich blood to all parts of our body, ensuring that our organs and tissues receive the nutrients and oxygen they need to function properly. At the same time, the heart receives impure, deoxygenated blood from the body's tissues and sends it to the lungs to be reoxygenated. This continuous cycle of giving and receiving is essential for our survival and is a testament to the heart's unselfish nature.

We spend much of time and effort in planning our professions and finances, but why don't we plan our physical fitness as well? If you are not scheduling the fitness your entire money plan become nonfunctional. You may not healthy enough to spend your hard-earned money. All that hard earned money will go to hospital ICU. Being fit is like being in love with yourself. Unless you love and respect your body, nobody else will. Of any kind of stress you have, being fit will guarantee that you waken up with a smile. Stress is unavoidable in life, being fit will help you get over your day without a painful body and an exhausted mind.

Regular exercise not only helps release tension and stress from the body, but it also triggers the body's natural parasympathetic response, allowing for rest, relaxation, and recuperation. Additionally, exercise stimulates the release of endorphins, which can positively affect mood and improve emotional clarity, concentration, relaxation, and sleep. By taking just ten to fifteen minutes of brisk exercise, any movement that increases heart rate and deepens breathing, you can give yourself an easy and positive boost when feeling less than your best.

If you are doing the exercise with suspicion of achieving the goal it will be like driving the car with one foot on the accelerator and other on the brake, you may make slight progress, you won't enjoy the journey and neither will around you. Being fit isn't a destination; it's an ongoing process of discovery. The discovery of what brings out the best in you. A misinformation with fitness seekers is, they've always looked at people who were athletic, thin, or visibly chiseled as fit, never dreaming that a positive state of mind and body are both by-products of becoming fit and actually a possibility in their lives.

The key to keeping weight off and staying healthy is activity. Scheduled exercise should be part of the program, but incorporating activity into your life every single day is the not-so-secret route to long-term success. "Positive impact on health" is not the same as "lean and fit," but it is a start or a supplement to a regular workout program.

Do you want to be fit to live a long, healthy life? You might want to see your grandchildren grow up, enjoy an active retirement, or avoid some of the health problems you see plaguing older relatives. Do you want to be fit to improve your love life? If you believe you haven't found a mate because of your appearance, if you fear your partner is losing interest because you've let yourself go, or if your spouse has left you for someone thinner, you might want to shape up for this most personal of reason.

The thin lean look is a media invention. There is range of body types and weights and what is healthy might be totally different than the next person". Is it possible to be both fat and fit? Yes, Two-hundred-kilogram sumo wrestlers, one twenty-kilogram football defensemen, and some long-distance or endurance swimmers are both strong and overweight. However, they cannot be described as completely fit. They are functionally fit for their chosen sports. For most people, balanced fitness leads to a long, healthy life. Being active rather than sedentary is the critical factor in health and longevity.

The universe we live in is characterized by movement and rhythm. When healthy, the organs in our body work together like a well-tuned orchestra, with the brain and nervous system acting as the conductor. Conversely, an unhealthy body can be out of tune and discordant.

When we get sick, it affects us more than anyone else. Doctors are not emotionally involved, and our family members only suffer to some degree. But we have to pay the bills, endure the pain, and depend on others for help. We can avoid this trauma by taking care of our health throughout our lives. We need to make consistent efforts until we die. Gandhi once said that he did not want to die of illness, because he had done everything, he could to stay healthy.

Today's world is full of opportunities. There is very high chance and opportunities to choose the good and bad. Choice is ours. Olden days the choices were limited. Everybody has undergone some sort of physical activity for their survival and food were natural and not adulterated. Today's world, the knowledge and understanding of proper choice is very important.

Just as there are five fingers in a palm, education has five main objectives, including physical, mental, social, intellectual, and emotional goals. Neglecting any of these components can impact our overall well-being, similar to how a broken spoke affects the stability of a cycle wheel. When the spokes are broken, the cycle wheel tend to bend when applying load on it, that is quite similar to our life. When we need to face the hard realities of life, going become difficult without wholesome development, through proper education. Unfortunately, physical activity is not always given adequate importance in our society or education system, leading to various psychosomatic disorders and diseases. However, taking walks in nature or engaging in physical activity can do wonders for our physical, emotional, and spiritual well-being. It's essential to focus on all components of wellness to achieve true personal development.

Long Term Physical Fitness

Maintaining a regular exercise routine can have a significant positive impact on your overall health and well-being. With 168 hours in a week, dedicating just 2.5 hours to exercise can help you stay healthy, happy, and disease-free. By spending 30 minutes a day for five days a week, you can keep your body in good physical condition and establish exercise as a way of life.

Exercise is not a quick fix to achieve your fitness goals, but it is a long-term investment in your health. As you make exercise a part of your daily routine, you not only improve your own physical and mental health, but you also inspire others to follow your lead and adopt a more positive way of life. One of the many benefits of exercise is its ability to reduce visceral fat, which can lead to a range of lethal diseases if left unchecked. Bring out the best version of you by engaging in regular physical activity.

Fitness is a personal and altruistic endeavor that benefits both oneself and loved ones. If given the choice, would you be willing to trade your current life for that of a bedridden billionaire with paralysis? Remember, imagination is like a muscle, and exercising it can lead to greater creativity. Thomas Edison, when asked about his 10,000 attempts to invent the incandescent bulb, famously replied that he had not failed but had discovered 10,000 ways how not to do it. Persistence is key in achieving and maintaining fitness goals, and the success requires overcoming the many tempting distractions along the way. Therefore, we must persist in our efforts to overcome these obstacles and stay focused on our fitness goals, while ensuring that our actions benefit both ourselves and those we care about.

Television advertisements and health magazine covers can be misleading and tempting with their attractive captions, such as "Walk Your Way to Fitness," "Cardio Quickie," and "Get Your Body Ready for the Beach." These messages may sound like quick solutions to achieving the perfect body, but in reality, they oversimplify the complex process of achieving fitness and may not be suitable for everyone.

It's important to remember that our bodies are not race cars that can be pushed to their limits without consequences. Expecting to go from sitting at a desk all day to powering through squats or cycling long distances in a short time is unrealistic and can even be harmful. It's crucial to start slowly, build a foundation of strength and endurance, and gradually increase intensity over time.

We should also be wary of advertisements that promote unrealistic body standards and suggest that certain body types are superior or more desirable. Fitness is about feeling healthy and strong, not conforming to societal beauty norms. We should focus on achieving realistic and sustainable fitness goals that prioritize our physical and mental well-being.

Overall, it's important to approach fitness with patience, dedication, and a long-term perspective. Rather than seeking quick fixes or following the latest fads, we should focus on building healthy habits that support our overall health and well-being.

Just like Rome was not built in a day, achieving fitness is a lifelong process rather than a short-term goal. When we exercise, we are essentially telling our bodies that we may not enjoy the present discomfort, but we will be grateful for the benefits it brings in the future.

The pain we experience during our workout today is the strength we will possess tomorrow. It is important to keep this in mind and push ourselves to keep going even when we feel like giving up. Sometimes, progress can be slow, but it's important to remember that every effort counts and eventually it will lead to success.

Drawing inspiration from a stonecutter who persists in hammering away at a rock, even if there is no visible progress for a prolonged period of time, can be valuable. With time and perseverance, the rock will eventually split into two with the final blow. It's worth noting that the stone does not break solely because of the last strike; it's due to the combined impact of all the previous hammer blows. Similarly, in fitness journey, it's crucial to keep moving forward and not give up, even if the results are not immediate or visible. Just like the stonecutter, persistence and consistency will ultimately bring fitness and happiness.

It may be risky to step out of our comfort zone, but it is necessary for growth. Our capacity to grow is directly related to how much we are willing to endure discomfort. By pushing ourselves to explore new challenges, we can continue to develop and evolve.

The human body's ability to walk on two legs might have led to instability to the spine and back pain. However, the arch of the foot provides four points of contact with the ground to stabilize the body during movement. The height variation among humans is mainly due to the difference in the length of leg bones. Interestingly, bone repair in the body is similar to maintaining a bridge. The bridge may remain open for repairs, but workers continue to work on it without passengers knowing. Similarly, bone repair and maintenance occur continuously in the body without disrupting daily activities.

To lose excess fat in the belly area, it is important to focus on overall weight loss. Spot reduction, or targeting a specific area for fat loss, is not possible through exercise alone. Attempting to lose belly fat through endless crunches can actually be detrimental to your health, causing strain on your back and abdomen.

Instead, it is important to focus on a healthy and balanced diet that promotes weight loss and a consistent exercise routine that engages the entire body. Similar to formatting the hard drive of a computer to remove a stubborn virus, focusing on overall health and fitness will ultimately lead to a reduction in belly fat and improved overall well-being.

Exercise and diet are indeed interconnected when it comes to achieving fitness goals. Exercise can be thought of as the bow, providing the strength and power to propel you towards your target, while diet can be considered the arrow, providing the necessary direction and precision. In the second chapter, the importance of diet in maintaining a healthy body has been explained.

The weakest link can be a hindrance to achieving the desired outcome. Stiff muscles and tendons are like the old, dried out rubber bands you find in the back of your desk drawer. Lack of stretching makes the muscles, tight like guitar strings. For example, a weak ligament or muscle tissue can lead to injury during exercise, or poor dietary choices can undermine the benefits of a consistent exercise routine. Therefore, it is important to pay attention to all aspects of fitness and address any weaknesses to ensure optimal results.

While it is true that muscle tissue is denser than fat and therefore weighs more per volume, the statement "muscle tissue is heavier than fat" can be misleading. It is more accurate to say that a kilogram of muscle takes up less space than a kilogram of fat. In terms of measuring fitness, weight loss can be an important indicator of progress, but it is not the only factor to consider. Body composition, including the ratio of muscle to fat, is also important. Measuring progress through changes in clothing size can be a useful alternative to solely relying on the scale.

The statement about surrounding oneself with those who are fatter to appear thinner is not a healthy or productive approach to fitness. It is important to focus on one's own individual progress and not compare oneself to others. Fitness should be about personal improvement and well-being, not about external validation or comparisons to others. The importance of mindset, avoiding comparison with others, finding joy in exercise, and recognizing the impact of physical fitness on overall health and productivity. They also suggest that taking care of oneself through exercise and a healthy lifestyle can have a positive impact not only on an individual level, but on society as a whole.

Consider the strength of your legs as being directly proportional to the engine power in your car. When your limbs are strong, your body can propel itself quickly, much like a powerful engine can make a car go faster. In the same way, our bodies can become more powerful through athleticism and physical fitness, which can be viewed as a new religion to follow. Starting with walking and progressing to jogging is similar to changing gears in a car. To begin a fitness program, it's best to start in first gear and gradually progress to higher gears over time.

There is a story about a wise man and a fool who were given a bowl each, with the task of collecting raindrops in them. The wise man immediately put his bowl out and collected a few drops every time it drizzled or rained. In contrast, the fool waited for the perfect time to collect the raindrops. As a result, the wise man's bowl was quickly filled while the fool continued to wait for the ideal moment. The lesson to be learned from this story is that there is no perfect time to begin exercising. Today is the best time to start and take the first step towards achieving your fitness goals.

Taking care of your health is like depositing money into a bank account, which will accumulate over time and pay dividends in the form of improved physical and mental health. However, if you neglect your health and only use your "health credit card" by relying on medical interventions and treatments when you get sick or injured, you may end up paying a much higher price in terms of lost productivity, reduced quality of life, and increased healthcare costs. By investing in your health through regular exercise, healthy eating habits, and other lifestyle changes, you can enjoy a better quality of life and avoid many preventable health problems.

As you begin your fitness journey, it's important to recognize that you are the leader in control of your life. Motivation should be seen as the overarching strategy in your pursuit of long-term fitness, while specific goals serve as the individual tactics you will employ to achieve success. In any battle, it is critical to know exactly what you're fighting for and to maintain a clear view of your objectives. Ultimately, you must remain focused on your goals to achieve lasting fitness.

The analogy of a master gardener applies to teaching yoga and exercises as well. Just as a master gardener knows how much water, fertilizer, and pruning a plant needs, an expert in yoga and exercise knows how to guide and teach their students without causing harm. It's important to avoid "pruning" our children or beginners in yoga and exercise, as we may inadvertently damage them in a way that cannot be undone. Therefore, it's important to seek out a knowledgeable and experienced teacher who can guide and support us on our journey towards fitness and wellness.

Exercising outdoors has numerous benefits for both the mind and body. The fresh air and natural daylight can have a positive impact on mood and overall well-being. Additionally, it's important to note that body temperature fluctuates throughout the day, with the lowest temperature typically occurring in the morning, peaking around midday, and then gradually decreasing again in the evening. Proper breathing techniques can also have a transformative effect on the body, improving overall strength and vitality.

Means and Methods for Fitness

The truth is that transforming yourself from a sedentary, out-of-shape person to someone fit is not instant. Many people think they can change their bodies quickly, but fitness and good health don't come about overnight. That should be no surprise. After all, we didn't add those extra pounds or become unfit overnight. Shaping up is a process that has to start with a few fundamental steps. Figure out where you are, set realistic goals, and try to determine how you can accomplish them. Then begin.

"Today is the first day of the rest of your life."

Outdoor exercise can have benefits beyond just the physical workout, such as exposure to natural sunlight, fresh air, and the opportunity to explore new environments. In contrast, gym workouts may be more controlled and predictable, but lack the variety and challenges of outdoor exercise. Riding a bike outdoors requires more coordination and balance than a stationary bike in the gym, as outdoor terrain can be uneven and unpredictable. This can engage more muscles and provide a more well-rounded workout.

Adding a Swiss ball to an office can provide a simple and effective way to incorporate physical activity into the workday. Using the ball for sitting or as a tool for exercise can improve posture, engage core muscles, and reduce the negative effects of prolonged sitting.

In order to achieve your fitness goals, it is important to avoid being like a lawyer or wicketkeeper, who are always appealing for different reasons. Instead, set your goals and work hard to achieve them. It is possible to live a life that is twenty-five years younger than your actual age. In the future, we may even see the emergence of airport exercise clubs, which would allow busy travelers to get a workout in between flights.

Whatever you do, most important is to take the first step, do that first push up, take the first reach to your toe, start that committed breathing, like most Indians who habitually take a bath with cold water a bucket would understand-it is like pouring the first mug on your head -once that is done -the rest follows on its own. So go ahead -pour that first mug- Run on the beach, take rock climbing classes, Roller skate, take up belly dancing. Learn to let go of your inhibitions and don't stop at your gym. Think fitness, think fun, think adventure, Think outside your gym.

It's important to remember that beauty is in the eye of the beholder. Don't worry about others' opinions and focus on being confident and happy with yourself. Keep your workout routine safe, simple, and smart by following the KISS principle (keep it simple and smart). Remember that every journey starts with a single step, so be your own boss and do what is right for you. Commit to yourself because you deserve it.

According to the Dalai Lama, to know what you have done in the past, look at your body, and to know what you will do in the future, look at your mind. So, instead of just focusing on grades, it's important to consider whether a child is getting enough active play, which can promote hormonal balance and overall health.

Take hold of today, for it is the only day you truly have. Yesterday has already passed and tomorrow is uncertain. However, if you live today to the fullest, with happiness and hope, yesterday will be remembered as a dream and tomorrow will be a vision of promise. So, cherish this day and make the most of it.

Surya Namaskar

Surya Namaskar is a powerful yoga practice that can transform your physical and mental wellbeing. It's like adding a pinch of salt to food, distinctly altering its taste. Stiffness in the body reflects mental rigidity and a lack of creativity. Ill health is often caused by an imbalance in the body's energy system. Surya Namaskar is like a daily health tonic that can inject prana, or life force, into your body's existing structures. The spine plays a crucial role in our overall health, serving as the link between the brain and the body. It's like the trunk of a tree, supporting the entire body structure. The top vertebra, which supports the skull, is known as the atlas, like the mythical figure Atlas who supported the earth upon his shoulders.

From an Ayurvedic point of view, everything is paired. We have a right and left side, hot and cold, sun and moon, masculine and feminine, sympathetic and parasympathetic nerves, stimulating and calming substances, a pair of eyes and ears, and the concept of yin and yang in Chinese philosophy, which represents darkness and brightness. Similarly, in our body, agonist and antagonist muscles work in a synchronized manner, where one muscle contracts while the other muscle relaxes. It is essential to maintain this balance in our muscles to achieve optimal health and wellbeing.

Ageing and Exercising

Aging is inevitable, but we can strive to age gracefully. It's important to have the mindset of wanting to die young, but at an old age. Many people believe that you can't teach an old dog new tricks, but it's never too late to start enjoying exercise. Consistency is crucial for fitness at any age, yet it's often neglected. When God called upon an aging Moses to lead the Israelites out of Egypt at the age of eighty, one can only imagine how he felt. Retirement shouldn't mean retiring from life, but rather retiring to something. In the Bible, there are numerous examples of older individuals being chosen for various duties, such as Joshua and Moses. God fulfilled his promise to Abraham of having a son at the age of one hundred, and Sarah gave birth to Isaac when she was around 90 years old.

Age is indeed just a number, as these playful expressions aptly demonstrate. At 47 years young, one might humorously claim to be "sweet seventeen with thirty years of experience." It's a delightful reminder that age is not a barrier to staying youthful at heart and in spirit. Moreover, the observation that dry fruits can be costlier than fresh fruits underscore the idea that value and vitality can transcend the years we've lived. Ultimately, what truly matters is the zest for life and the willingness to embrace each day with enthusiasm, regardless of the number associated with our age. Adaptability is the essential ingredient for a successful life in later years, as the generation gap often creates differences between younger and older individuals.

Senior citizens should keep their brains stimulated, just as they do their other bodily muscles. Activities with low light intensity and indoor games are advisable for them. Playing chess and solving puzzles are great ways to activate the brain and prevent memory loss.

The concept of a one-size-fits-all approach in fitness training implies that everyone can achieve their fitness goals through the same routine or program. However, this approach is ineffective because every individual has unique physical abilities, health conditions, and fitness goals. Fitness training should be tailored to the individual's specific needs and goals to achieve the desired results. For example, an older adult may need to focus on mobility and stability exercises, while a young athlete may need to prioritize strength and power development. Moreover, even within the same age group, there can be significant variations in body composition, fitness level, and health status, which further emphasizes the need for personalized fitness training programs.

If you notice the oil indicator in your car is low, it can still travel a few more kilometers without issue. Similarly, during a workout, pushing through fatigue to complete a few more repetitions can help increase your potential. These additional repetitions, made despite tiredness, can lead to improvement and positive adaptation. Exercise can mainly induce following benefits to the aged people.

- Improved cardiovascular health: Exercise helps to maintain healthy blood pressure and cholesterol levels, reducing the risk of heart disease and stroke.

- Enhanced muscular strength and balance: Regular physical activity can help to prevent falls and fractures, and improve overall mobility and independence.

- Reduced risk of chronic diseases: Exercise has been linked to a lower risk of developing chronic conditions such as type 2 diabetes, arthritis, and certain types of cancer.

- Improved mental health: Physical activity has been shown to reduce symptoms of depression and anxiety, as well as improve cognitive function and overall mood.

- Increased social interaction: Group exercise classes or activities can provide opportunities for social interaction and help to combat loneliness and social isolation.

Overall, regular exercise is essential for maintaining good health and wellbeing in aged people.

Strength training

People are often inspired to exercise during the Olympics and the World Cup, but persistence is lacking. The registration fee is the primary source of income for many fitness centers. Continuity in practice is very rare after the initial motivation wanes. Jokingly, we say that the gym is the only place where we have to work and pay.

Weight training can be a great mood booster for human being, but it's important to approach it safely to avoid injury. Unfortunately, some may feel pressure to lift heavier weights than they can handle, leading to strains, sprains, and other injuries. It's important to remember that proper form and gradual progression are key to a safe and effective weight training routine.

The state of our health is fragile, much like a palace made out of a deck of cards. Any alteration or disruption can cause the entire structure to collapse. It's important to take care of ourselves, especially when it comes to exercising. Going to the gym on an empty stomach not only leads to poor performance but also increases the risk of injuries such as sprains, strains, and muscle pulls.

Treat your body like it's not yours, treat it's somebody else's and you have it on rent for a while. It's like if I give you my car, you would drive it at least ten times more carefully than how you drive your car. Drive it slower over speed breakers, return it with full petrol tank, have the right amount of air in the tyres, not jump signals etc.

Our body is a wonderful creation of God. It has all the software pre-installed, which can be used to reboot ourselves, whenever in need. Only you have to be literate enough to operate this machine, called human body. Our body is like following river. The cells o four body are constantly getting replaced with new ones throughout our life.

Pace Yourself or Push Yourself?

We are all familiar with the fable of the hare and the tortoise, where the hare begins the race with a burst of energy, but gets easily distracted and eventually loses to the slow and steady tortoise who never loses sight of the finish line. When it comes to starting a workout routine, many people have good intentions but tend to act like hares. They sign up for long gym memberships or buy expensive home equipment, and start working out frantically to make up for lost time. However, their enthusiasm wanes quickly and they often quit within two months. This can be due to injuries, exhaustion, boredom, or simply not being prepared for the long-term commitment. The key is to be like the tortoise, steadily building your fitness routine and making it a consistent part of your daily life.

Beyond the Comfort Zone

Exercise experts have conducted numerous studies to determine the most effective type and intensity of exercise to burn fat. While there is still some debate, many experts now believe that high-intensity interval training (HIIT) is one of the most effective methods. This involves alternating periods of intense activity with periods of rest or low-intensity activity. HIIT has been shown to burn more calories and fat than steady-state cardio exercise, such as jogging on a treadmill for an extended period of time.

However, it's important to note that the most effective type and intensity of exercise will vary from person to person. Factors such as age, fitness level, and health conditions can all impact what type of exercise is best for an individual. It's important to consult with a healthcare professional or certified fitness trainer to create a workout plan that is tailored to your specific needs and goals.

After you get into workout mode, it's important to keep pushing yourself to reach your goals. If you get to a certain point in your program and don't increase the challenge and/or duration, it's like putting your car into cruise control. You'll make a journey, but you won't be revving up the engine. Exercise experts have long agreed that revving up the engine is important in getting leaner and fitter, but there have been long-running debates about what type of exercise and what intensity are the most effective at burning fat. Settlement of this issue is on the way.

One thing that is clear is that exercise intensity plays a significant role in burning fat. High-intensity interval training (HIIT) has gained popularity in recent years as a highly effective method for burning fat and improving overall fitness. HIIT involves short bursts of high-intensity exercise followed by brief recovery periods. This type of training not only burns calories during the workout but also increases the body's metabolic rate, which leads to continued fat burning even after the workout is over.

Learn to listen to your body

Fitness is not just about following a set program or routine. It requires understanding and listening to your body. In the beginning, it can be difficult to differentiate between good and bad pain, exhaustion and pushing yourself to the limit. However, with time and practice, you will learn to understand the signals your body sends you. You will know when you need to rest and when you need to push yourself harder. You will also understand how to warm up and stretch effectively to prevent injuries. This understanding will also help you develop the discipline needed to stick to your fitness regimen. When you start missing your workouts, your body will let you know that it's missing something. By developing this sense, you'll know that you're on the right track to becoming fitter and healthier.

Recovery

The story of the two woodcutters serves as a reminder of the importance of taking a break after a workout. One of the woodcutters worked tirelessly without taking any breaks, while the other took regular breaks every hour. Surprisingly, the woodcutter who took breaks managed to cut more wood than his counterpart. When asked about the secret to his success, the second woodcutter revealed that during his breaks, he would sharpen his axe, which made his work more efficient and effective.

Similarly, after a workout, it is essential to allow the body to rest and recover. Taking a break and allowing the body to recuperate will enable you to perform better during your next workout. It's like sharpening your axe so that you can cut more wood in less time. Without rest, the body becomes fatigued, and you may end up doing more harm than good. Therefore, it is crucial to make rest and recovery an integral part of your fitness routine.

Mental fitness

In modern world physical exhaustion has been replaced by mental fatigue. Competitive, consumeristic, capitalistic modern life putting stain on mental fabric, resulting in mental health disorders in most part of the world. If we go by the principle of cause and effect, every thought is a cause and our health is an effect. Necessary to take charge of our thoughts. We need to have a blueprint for our goal. Then you will be on auto mode and will not have consciously effort into it. The hardest part is getting your mind in shape, rest is easy. The first and greatest victory, is to conquer self. "A good coach trains your body. A great coach trains your mind as well". The mind is like a curtain between you and your true self. It is like a dust between you and your mirror. Meditation is like a gym in which you develop the powerful mental muscles.

Performance is the function of mind and body coordination-which comes from repetition and practice of the particular activity. Arnold Schwarzenegger definitely has stronger arms than Shoaib Akhtar, but can he throw the ball as fast? The sunflower follows the sun across the sky because an inner mechanism controls that behavior, and on cloudy days the mechanism automatically shows the intelligence of not to operate, such as our mind in the body.

Man is a social animal and lack of social connectivity is detrimental to emotional wellbeing and even heart health. Always keep this imaginary dustbin next to you, and throw away all unwanted emotions and things. Engaging in sports, games, and fitness activities can undoubtedly serve as a powerful tool for enhancing mental well-being. The everyday experiences of both winning and losing in these pursuits help children adapt to the reality of life's small setbacks without being overwhelmed. In today's digital age, social media sets exceedingly high expectations and often leaves individuals dissatisfied, particularly affecting the younger generation and their mental health. It has become increasingly common to find mental health experts in schools and colleges. Fortunately, physical activities offer an effective antidote to these challenges. In the realm of sports and games, participants experience holistic development, impacting their physical, mental, social, intellectual, and emotional dimensions, thus contributing to their overall well-being.

Stress

To achieve success in life, one must be prepared to face various obstacles that could distract them from their goal. Stress is one of the few things that seem to be permanent in our lives. However, it is important to not let these obstacles and distractions hinder our progress towards the finish line. It is comparable to a potter who must work hard to make the clay malleable by kneading, slapping, patting, and caressing it with the right amount of pressure at the right time to ensure that the pot becomes useful. Similarly, just as we cannot control the tides of the ocean or the seasons, we cannot change the nature of our individual bodies. There are no quick fixes in life, and we must be willing to put in the effort required to achieve our goals. This is like building a tunnel that is hundreds of meters long - even at the 99th meter, with only one more meter to go until the end, the light is not yet visible. Therefore, to succeed, one must persevere and continue to push forward until they reach the end.

Stress is a part of daily life, and it can have a profound effect on our bodies. An excellent example of this is holding a glass of water in one hand for an extended period. Initially, it seems effortless, but as time passes, the hand muscles begin to tire, making it difficult to maintain the same position. Similarly, if we allow stress to build up without taking any measures to alleviate it, it can take a toll on our bodies and minds. If stress continues to accumulate, it can lead to fatigue, loss of creativity, and decreased enthusiasm towards life.

Therefore, it is essential to find ways to manage stress as early as possible. One effective way is to participate in sports or games, which can help reduce stress and provide a healthy outlet for physical and mental energy. Engaging in physical activity can significantly reduce the production of the stress hormone cortisol, as the positive hormones released during exercise have the ability to counterbalance the negative effects of cortisol. By taking proactive steps to manage stress, we can protect our bodies and minds from the harmful effects of chronic stress and enjoy a healthier, more fulfilling life.

Depression

Russian space program recognized the importance of exercise in space to help prevent depression and other negative effects of spaceflight on the human body. In fact, the Soviet Union was the first to recognize the importance of exercise in space, and they developed a special stationary bicycle for cosmonauts to use while in orbit. Later, they also developed a treadmill for use on space missions. Research has shown that regular exercise can help prevent the physical and psychological effects of long-term spaceflight, including muscle atrophy, bone loss, cardiovascular changes, and depression. Exercise can also help astronauts maintain their physical and mental health during missions, and improve their overall quality of life in space.

Exercise can lead to the release of certain chemicals in the brain called catecholamines, which can have a positive effect on mood and help alleviate symptoms of depression. These chemicals include dopamine, norepinephrine, and epinephrine, which are neurotransmitters that play a role in regulating mood, attention, and arousal.

However, it's important to note that exercise alone may not be sufficient to treat clinical depression, and it should not be used as a substitute for professional medical treatment. Exercise can be a helpful component of a comprehensive treatment plan for depression, along with other interventions such as therapy, medication, and lifestyle changes. It's always best to consult with a healthcare professional for personalized recommendations for managing depression.

Happiness

By investing just Rs. 3000 in an exercise cycle, one could potentially save up to Rs. 300000 on a coronary bypass surgery. This highlights the importance of taking care of our health and wellbeing, as prevention is often more effective and cost-efficient than treatment. Furthermore, laughter is said to be the best medicine - it is like internal jogging that can have a positive impact on our physical and mental health. It has been proven that laughing regularly can reduce stress levels also. Therefore, taking the time to lighten up, laugh, and play can have significant benefits for our overall health and longevity. As the saying goes, he who laughs, lasts, and laugh lines may even lengthen our lifelines.

Spirituality

The sounds described in our scriptures like Aum, Amen, Allah, Hmmm. Humming a mantra create vibration of frequency of 432 hz. Which is the natural frequency of the universe. When we practice it, our cells also start vibrating with that frequency and bring health and happiness in our life. Faith is like a muscle. The more you exercise it, the stronger it gets. The less you use it, the more it shrinks. Therefore, taking care of our emotional and physical health is crucial to our overall well-being. Practicing stress-reducing activities, such as meditation and exercise, and cultivating positive emotions, such as love and compassion, can help promote heart health and improve our overall quality of life.

Spirituality can play a significant role in helping individuals achieve success, especially in sports and games. Here are ten reasons why spirituality is crucial for success in sports and games:

1. Spirituality provides individuals with a sense of purpose and meaning, which can motivate them to achieve their goals in sports and games.

2. It helps individuals develop mental toughness, enabling them to handle the pressures and challenges that come with competing at a high level.

3. It helps individuals cultivate a positive attitude, which can enhance their performance and increase their chances of success.

4. Spirituality can help individuals develop a deep sense of gratitude, allowing them to appreciate their abilities, opportunities, and achievements.

5. It provides individuals with a sense of inner peace, which can help them stay focused and calm in high-pressure situations.

6. It can help individuals develop a sense of empathy, allowing them to understand and connect with their teammates and opponents better.

7. Spirituality can help individuals develop resilience, enabling them to bounce back from setbacks and failures.

8. It can help individuals develop a sense of humility, allowing them to acknowledge their weaknesses and work towards improving themselves.

9. It helps individuals develop a sense of discipline, which can enhance their ability to focus and stay committed to their goals.

10. Spirituality can help individuals develop a sense of interconnectedness, allowing them to see how their actions and achievements can impact others positively.

In conclusion, spirituality can be a powerful tool for individuals looking to succeed in sports and games. By developing a strong spiritual practice, individuals can cultivate the mindset and qualities necessary to achieve their goals and lead fulfilling, meaningful lives.

Home Based Fitness Programme

Maintaining a healthy body weight is important for overall health, and exercising regularly is a great way to achieve that. However, going to the gym may not be possible or affordable for everyone. The good news is that there are many items available that can be used as home fitness equipment at a cheap rate, such as an Ab wheel, skipping rope, soup cans, plastic bottles filled with water or sand, gym ball, dumbbells, and a pull-up bar that can be fixed on the wall. With these items, you can do exercises for all the muscles in your body.

Creating a home workout program is an excellent way to achieve perfect fitness, and it can be done by accumulating activities for the final goal. Competitions among family members can be introduced to make the program more interesting. For example, during a game show, family members can guess the answer, and those who get the correct answer can demand an activity for other members, such as 5 push-ups, 20 sit-ups, 5 burpees, etc. During family time, when watching a favorite program, they can choose a particular character, and when that actor appears, all family members have to perform a specific activity, such as plank, one leg stand, free squat, etc.

Home workouts offer the convenience of being able to read or watch TV while exercising. Walking on a treadmill and watching TV or browsing the internet is also possible. The climatic conditions or costumes are not a hindrance to home workouts. Even with 5 minutes, you can perform 10 Surya namaskars, which will enhance oxygenated blood flow to the brain and help you feel relaxed. This habit can be continued while traveling, as a hotel room is enough to do your fitness activities. In rural areas, the branches of trees are a better option for pull-ups and related activities. Partner stretching and carrying one person over the other are also activities that can be performed in a home setting.

While doing such activities, it is essential to take care of proper form and include variety in your program to maintain a balance among your muscles. After a heavy workout, it is essential to warm down by laying down on the floor to improve venous return and speedy recovery. In summary, home workouts offer a convenient and cost-effective way to achieve perfect fitness, and with the right equipment and program, you can achieve your fitness goals without going to the gym.

Make Fitness a Habit

Exercise and physical activity can be very effective in preventing many chronic diseases such as heart disease, diabetes, and obesity. In addition, regular exercise can also help prevent injuries by improving balance, flexibility, and muscle strength. It is important for healthcare providers to encourage their patients to adopt a healthy lifestyle that includes regular physical activity and movement, rather than just treating them when they are already sick or injured. This can help prevent many health problems before they even start, leading to better overall health and wellbeing. By spreading the fever of fitness, we can initiate a revolution that has the potential to lower medical expenses, increase productivity at work, bless us with a longer lifespan, and bring immense satisfaction by positively influencing the lives of others. If each of us takes responsibility for spreading the message of fitness and encourages others to adopt healthy lifestyles, we can collectively create a healthier and happier world. Through this movement, we can inspire people to prioritize their well-being and help them understand the benefits of fitness beyond just physical health. As more and more individuals embrace fitness as a way of life, we can create a ripple effect that transforms communities and ultimately leads to a healthier and happier world.

However, it's important to remember that the most effective workout program is one that is tailored to your specific goals, abilities, and preferences. Consult with a qualified fitness professional to design a program that works for you and your body. And remember, consistency is key. Keep pushing yourself, but also listen to your body and adjust your program as necessary to avoid injury or burnout.

According to John Basedow, the windshield of a car is designed to be big and open, allowing for a clear view of the road ahead. This is because what lies in front of us is often more important than what is behind us. The future holds endless possibilities and opportunities for growth, and it is crucial to focus on that. On the other hand, the rear-view mirror is much smaller in comparison, as it is meant to provide only a brief glimpse of what's behind us. While our past experiences can provide valuable lessons, it is not healthy to dwell on them or let them define our present or future. We must learn to let go of the past and move forward with a positive outlook towards the future.

Fitness is the fruit of effort, not daydreams. Result will speak for themselves, so bury the past. You have made mistakes, that's alright, you are just human. Stop saying one day I will be fit. Stay on the course; come what may. Embrace a positive addiction to physical activity, as this habit is often the key to success in life; just as a fish thrives in water, strive to incorporate physical activity into your daily plans wherever you go.

Finally, physical activity is so essential to our health that if it could be packaged into a pill, it would be the next blockbuster drug. Incorporating regular exercise into our daily routine can have a profound impact on our overall health and well-being, making it a vital component of a healthy lifestyle.

Points to remember

- Workouts focused on acquiring a six pack or muscle popping out of your T-shirt might not be for you. Avoid the common outside in approach to fitness. If you do not have general fitness and directly going for hard weight training to enlarge your muscles is like spending lot of time to decorate your house before fixing the leaking roof through which water is sweeping onto your bed. Become aware of fitness before registering in a gymnasium or buying aerobic equipment's to make your body as your favorite models or film stars.

- Adopt the "inside-out" approach to both fitness and wellness. Firstly, try to assess your current fitness level with the help of an expert. If you are obese or have a chronic back problem or high blood pressure or extreme stiffness or weakness on certain muscle groups then you take charge of your health, you should prioritize fixing these first before moving on to other superficial fitness goals.

- The right way to start is with holistic exercises like yoga postures and walking, and then move on to free hand fitness exercises like jogging, push-ups and free hand weights. The attainment of basic fitness is essential to go for high intensity and greater volume in practice.

- Even if you are walking, after walking at an easy pace sometime increase the pace and let your heart rate go up a bit. Walk up an incline once in a while to push yourself further. Even if you wish to practice yoga postures, after doing the asana easy for you, attempt some asana that are difficult and try to perfect them.

- Any exercise which doesn't increase the heart rate will not make much effect to the internal system. Walk the way people walk at busy railway stations to catch the train. Just do not walk too slowly or you might miss the train of getting into shape!

- Wake up stretches are good to activate the spine. Watch the animals like cat or dog immediately after waking up they go for some stretching exercises before going for the day. Likewise human beings also need some preparation before starting the daily routine. Light stretching after waking up from the bed is good to have energetic body throughout the day.

- You might have noticed that you get headaches in buses, crowded or smoke-filled places, centrally air-conditioned places like malls, aircraft etc. These congested places reduce the oxygen supply to the brain through blood flow, and causes headache. So, select well-ventilated and nature friendly places for exercise.

- While picking up things from the floor, especially heavy objects, always bend your knees to initially make use of leg muscles and hand muscles, otherwise the maximum strain on the back.
- While working on the health clubs avoid loud music, so that you can listen more to your body. A good warm-up reduces the chances of injury. Mobilizes the joints and producing heat to the muscles, resultantly muscles are ready for the activity. Activity is like driving car, it's good to start the engine and let the car heat up for few seconds, then you put it in the first gear, then the second, third, and fourth before going at very high speed.
- The slight pain or difficulty after the exercise we call "Sweet pain" because this is the stage of adaptation, which the positive changes are happening in our body.
- Hormones secreted during the exercise like Dopamine, Serotonin, Oxytocin, Endorphins which are known as happy hormone induces positive mood.
- Fitness is your cheapest health insurance. It has been realized that fitness adds not only years to one's life but life to one's years. Contradictory part of the modern world is that few are running to reduce the size of the stomach and many are running to fill the stomach. Fitness passionate can get maximum return in his life to any insurance bond can offer.
- Fitness Starts with Setting Goals -Would you plan a dinner party without a menu or recipes? Would you head out on a vacation without an itinerary and some maps? When you decide that

now is the time to get fit, set some goals for yourself at the outset. Be realistic and make them achievable Instead of dreaming about the unachievable body, think about improving, not perfecting, the body you have. Here are some examples of goals you can set:

1. You can set general goals such as slimming down, trimming your belly, toning your thighs, or building your upper torso in relation to your body now.

2. It is even more effective to set a specific goal such as losing 5 kilograms, going down two sizes, or fitting into an outfit you outgrew five years ago.

3. You can set an exercise goal such as being able to do 25 pushups, bench press 25 kg. Sustain an hour on a stationary bike or treadmill.

4. You can set a functional goal such as running or walking in a race, hiking up a high mountain, or refereeing your child's soccer game without practically collapsing till the final score is posted.

5. You can set a health goal such as reducing your blood pressure or lowering your cholesterol level.

6. You can set a scheduling goal such as working out at least three but preferably four times a week for a month or every other day until you've used up every session on a membership card at the gym.

7. You can sign up for a class that runs for a certain number of weeks and see it through such as a beginner weight-training course, a low-impact aerobics course, a water fitness course, a beginning yoga class, or planned walking sessions with a coach.

8. Think "trim" instead of "thin" -Think "healthy" instead of "skinny." Think "health "instead of "fashion." These are the thoughts you should keep in mind when embarking on a fitness or weight-loss program.

9. Exercise and weight- The exercise helps control weight. Scientists, nutritionists, and physiologists studying the relationship between diet and exercise have drawn conclusions that point to exercise as a weight-loss enhancer, not a detractor. When you exercise, you build muscle and become both fitter and leaner. "Tune Up That Muscle Machine."Make the core of it a workout log, which is like an exercise diary.

➢ Warm Up, Cool Down-The warm-up at the beginning of a workout and the cool-down afterward has a couple of things in common. Both involve relatively gentle movements and some stretching. The purpose of both the warm-up and the cool-down is to enhance flexibility, minimize discomfort, and even prevent injury. The warm-up specifically prepares the muscular system for the harder work to come. It helps you loosen up before your aerobic workout to get the blood flowing and to loosen your muscles for the upcoming exercises. The cool-down allows your body to relax, to discard some of the waste products and lactic acid you might have accumulated, and to return to a resting state after you are finished. If you are planning to walk or run, do a few hundred yards at a slower walk or a gentle jog. Start an aerobics routine with a few minutes of light, dance-like motions to bring your heart-rate up slowly and gradually. This warm-up period is vital in increasing the blood flow to your muscles, which in turn makes muscles and connective tissue more elastic. Before you enter into your routine, do a few gentle calf, hamstring, and hip flexor stretches to limber up. The cool-down routine is similar, but in reverse slowing the pace from your aerobic walk, run, or choreographed routine to enable your heart rate to return to fewer than 100 beats per minute. Soon, your breathing and heart rates will return to normal. Your Post-aerobic stretches can be stronger, because muscles are more elastic after a workout than before. Done over time, these stretches help lengthen the muscles and make you more flexible.

- What to Expect from Weight Training -Milo's story teaches us an important lesson about how to build strength and muscle. The key is to start with a manageable weight and gradually increase it over time. Milo began by lifting a small calf and continued to do so every day until the calf grew into a full-grown bull. This gradual increase in weight allowed Milo to build strength and muscle without causing injury or strain to his body. The same principles can be applied to strength training today. It's important to start with a weight that you can handle and gradually increase it as you become stronger. This gradual progression allows your muscles to adapt and grow over time, leading to increased strength and muscle mass.

- Remember that muscle is denser than fat, so a toned body looks slimmer, stronger, and more attractive than a flabby one. Also remember that a toned, slimmer-looking body might actually weigh as much as, or even more than, a flabby, out-of-shape one. For muscles to become stronger, you need to demand more of them than their usual workload. Working them harder in this way is known as overloading that's what you want to do when weight-training. Physiologically, when you lift enough weight to overload your muscles, you cause tiny tears in the muscle fibers. When they regenerate, the muscles become incrementally stronger. Not only will you be able to lift more in the gym, everyday activities will quickly become easier. In addition to the benefit of muscular strength in and of itself, strong muscles and strong bones are linked. As you build your muscles, your bones become stronger as a response to the greater force being exerted on them. In a sense, your bones try to "match" your muscles. You can help the process by taking in sufficient calcium and by participating in aerobic activities.

- Various studies indicate that weight training reduces various serious health risks. Strength training improves glucose metabolism, for example, which can help control adult-onset diabetes. Such training also helps speed the digestive process, or gastrointestinal transit time, and reduces the risk of colon cancer. It can help ease lower back pain and can reduce arthritis pain. Strength training can even help emotional well-being.

- A recent report in Medicine and Science in Sports and Fitness revealed that male and female volunteers experienced "significantly reduced anxiety" for three hours after a single weight-training session. The bad news about muscles is that, when they are not used, they lose strength rapidly. The good news, however, is that strength can easily and quickly be recaptured, even by people who have never worked with weights. Muscle tissue burns calories much faster than fat tissue, so even after you've stopped exercising for the day, the "furnace" muscles keep utilizing calories. In other words, strong muscles actually will raise your metabolism. Obviously, the best thing you can do for yourself is not let your muscles become weak and loose in the first place. If you are out of shape, be encouraged by the fact that muscles begin to build extremely quickly when you commence strength training.

- Feel Good About Feeling Sore -When you start a workout program that includes weight training, you can expect to feel sore and tired afterward. You might wonder whether you are doing yourself a favor or actually harming yourself. Keep in mind that, if you have not done anything like this, light weights and modest repetitions are the smart way to start. If you have not been doing any weight training and especially if your daily routine includes lifting nothing heavier than a cereal box you will feel sore. This is good because it means your muscles are being used.

- Women Need Weight Work, Too- Women, who are significantly more likely to suffer bone loss, weakness, and fractures later in life, need weight training even more than men. For women, osteoporosis should be the scariest word in the English language. Osteoporosis is serious bone loss that comes with age, inactivity, and calcium depletion. Beginning at about age 35, an adult woman can lose 1 percent of her bone mass every year, which translates to 5 to 7 pounds per decade. During and after menopause, a woman's muscle loss speeds up. Women who begin strength training replace fat with lean muscle. As you work out, you actually will find that you become more toned and slimmer from strength training, even if the number on the scale doesn't drop.

- Trimmers and Toners from TV to You-Cable television is flooded with infomercials for specialty items to help you trim or tone this body part or that. Such devices have been around for years, but seductive television infomercials, often with celebrity endorsements, fill them with an in-your-face presence that makes them hard to ignore. Many of the products hawked on television also are available at discount stores, sporting goods retailers, and perhaps even supermarkets. Some products are powerful and decently built; others are weak and marginally effective at best. It's hard to tell on the TV screen, and most people just thrust purchasing mistakes away rather than take advantage of the money-back guarantees that usually are part of the offers. If a product seduces you, try to take a good look at a real sample and evaluate its quality in relation to its price. You can always go home and order it, or you can buy it locally, perhaps even on sale. If you buy from a local retailer, you won't have to pay the dreaded shipping and handling add-on, and if you are unhappy with the product or it doesn't live up to its claims, you're more likely to return it to a local retailer than mail it back to a distant company. You will also find that such items are often available at garage sales, because many people order them but never use them.

- Other Paths to Stretching and Toning with Yoga -Yoga, a ritualized discipline, is as spiritual as it is physical. It is a versatile discipline that strengthens and tones the body, calms the mind, increases flexibility, and enhances introspection. It has even been called the world's oldest stress-management system. This ancient holistic philosophy from India now has as many branches as a cotton wood tree. Some are ancient traditions; others were founded more recently by modern masters. Although yoga is the foundation of a total lifestyle for some people, it is part of a fitness program for millions of others. In fact, many stretches now commonly used by athletes are yoga poses.

- The approximate daily step count for sedentary individuals is between 2000 to 4000 steps, which can be achieved through daily routines and household chores. Walking at a moderate pace for 30 minutes can add 2500 to 3000 steps to the total count. By gradually increasing the daily step count by 500 steps, individuals can aim to reach the target of 10000 steps for true fitness. Walking 10 thousand steps in a day is a good workout to attain perfect fitness. It is important to complement this daily walking routine with light strengthening and stretching exercises. This routine can be incorporated into office hours as well. To track progress, individuals can use a pedometer application on their smart phone or wear a smart watch that displays the total steps covered in a day. This way, they can monitor their progress and feel the satisfaction of achieving their goals, akin to paying for silver but receiving diamonds in return.

- The human body comprises over 600 muscles, and engaging in the same exercise routine every day may not activate all of them. Therefore, it is essential to incorporate variety in physical activities. Participating in different sports and workouts can activate all the muscles, ligaments, and tendons, significantly reducing the risk of injury and preventing boredom from setting in. Opting for different venues and teammates can also provide a refreshing experience. It is advisable to make changes to the workout routine, equipment, and practice location as much as possible.

- Isometrics: Icing for the Fitness Cake with ball-Fitness can be a whole new ball game with a big, inflated, rubber sphere called a fit ball or Swiss ball. Developed by Swiss physical therapists to help patients regain strength, balance, and flexibility, the fit ball makes a workout both productive and fun.

- Educate Yourself-No muscle group causes more agony and concern than the abdominals (or abs). Everyone wants them to be firm and flat. When it is really toned so that every muscular ripple shows, it is called washboard abs. Men like to build shapely pecs, and women who work their pecs often find that their breasts appear firmer and sometimes larger.

The early years of life are an optimal period for establishing healthy habits, such as consuming nutritious food and engaging in physical fitness. Unfortunately, many schools do not prioritize physical activity and instead focus solely on academics. Entrance tests for schools typically do not have a physical component, and anything that takes away from academic performance is often seen as a distraction to be avoided at all costs. However, this mindset needs to change in order to promote overall health and well-being among students. By prioritizing physical activity and creating environments that encourage movement, we can help prevent obesity and improve the overall health of our communities.

The saying "as you sow, so you reap" rings true when it comes to fitness. There are no shortcuts or quick fixes on the journey to good health - one must put in the necessary effort to see results. No magic pill exists that can substitute for hard work. However, for those with a strong willpower, there is always a way to achieve their goals. Every human being has been blessed with immense potential, and with persistence and continuous effort, anything is possible. So, if you have the determination and discipline to put in the work, success is within your grasp.

The famous saying "you sow a thought; you reap an action" holds true when it comes to physical fitness. The first step towards achieving a healthy body is to have a positive mindset and believe in yourself. This positive thought will lead to taking the necessary actions, such as following a balanced diet and engaging in regular exercise. Over time, these actions become habitual, and a healthy lifestyle is ingrained into one's character. This new character then shapes one's destiny, leading to a fulfilling and prosperous life.

On the other hand, negative thoughts can lead to detrimental actions, habits, and ultimately a negative destiny. It's crucial to pay attention to one's thoughts and strive to cultivate a positive mindset towards physical fitness. It's never too late to make a change, and by starting with a positive thought, anyone can achieve their health and fitness goals. So, take the first step today and sow a positive thought towards your physical fitness journey. It is important to take responsibility for our own happiness and well-being, rather than blaming others for our lack of motivation or discipline. The phrase "Altitude determines our attitude" emphasizes the impact of our mindset and perspective on our actions and outcomes, and highlights the importance of maintaining a positive and determined attitude towards our goals.

The sayings "a rolling stone gathers no moss" and "those who practice daily can lift elephants" are highly applicable to achieving optimal physical fitness through daily exercise. We all can do and let us put all our efforts to remain healthy throughout our life to make this world more livable. The miracle drug without any side effect is exercise. Exercise is preventive medicine and it needs to be a daily ritual just like brushing your teeth. Exercise is known as nature's antidepressant. You can't pour from an empty cup. Take care of yourself first. Be fit at first, then only you can make others fit. There are many people to talk but less number to act. Action speaks louder than voice is very relevant. Although the tree falls in the last cut, there is a lot of effort behind it, so don't expect immediate results in fitness practice. With patience and constant effort, it is certain that we can reach our desired fitness level.

Achieving fitness is a journey that requires patience and persistence. It's like digging a well - you may put in a lot of effort and dig deep, but if you don't reach the source of water, all that work will go to waste. Similarly, if you expect to see immediate results in your fitness journey, you may become discouraged and give up before reaching your goal.

With dedication and perseverance, you can achieve your fitness goals. Just remember to stay committed to the process and trust that your hard work will pay off in the end. Don't give up on your journey - the reward of a healthier and happier life is worth the effort.

Engaging in fitness activities serves as a silent role model for the younger generation, inspiring them to embrace a healthy lifestyle. It is, without a doubt, a form of social service, for as the saying goes, service to humanity is akin to service to God. In the realm of sports and fitness, there are no divisions of caste, creed, or politics. Simply by donning sports attire and participating, we unknowingly motivate many. A healthy populace is an invaluable asset to any nation, while weakness becomes a burden. It's fair to say that achieving proper physical fitness is not just a way of life, but life itself. So, let us embark on our journey of social service today.

> ***"When health is absent, wisdom cannot reveal itself, art cannot manifest, strength cannot fight, wealth becomes useless, and intelligence cannot be applied"***
>
> –**Herophilus** (Father of anatomy)

2

Nutrition

"He who has health has hope, and he who has hope has everything."

–Arabian Proverb

Modernization and the use of electronic equipment have made our lives easier and more convenient, but they have also made us more sedentary and have contributed to the rise of obesity and early onset of diseases such as diabetes. In addition, we have become more reliant on processed foods and have stopped cultivating our own food, leading to an increased use of pesticides and other harmful chemicals in our diet. Interestingly, the paradoxical situation arises with the use of preservatives and pesticides in the food supply chain. For example, fishermen catch fish and keep a portion for their own consumption without any added poison, but add preservatives to the portion for sale. Similarly, farmers separate their yield, keeping a portion without any poison for their own use, but add pesticides to the portion for sale. This results in a situation where people living in coastal areas end up eating poisoned vegetables, while those living in hilly areas end up consuming poisoned fish. This is a dangerous situation, as these harmful chemicals can have serious health implications and lead to various diseases. It's important to be mindful of our food choices and to support sustainable farming practices that prioritize the health of both people and the environment.

Supermarkets are designed to encourage customers to buy more products than they initially intended. This is known as "impulse buying" and can be influenced by various techniques used by supermarkets. For example, providing a basket instead of a small shopping cart can make customers feel like they need to fill the basket, leading to more purchases. Products for children are placed at their eye level to attract them, and essential commodities are kept at the end of the store to make customers walk through the entire store, increasing the chances of making additional purchases.

In addition, there is typically no clock or window in the store to make customers lose track of time and stay longer, and chocolates and other tempting items are often placed near the payment area to encourage impulse purchases. To avoid falling prey to these tactics, it is important to stick to a shopping list and avoid purchasing items that are not necessary. By being aware of these techniques, customers can make more informed decisions when shopping and avoid spending more than they intended.

The human body can be compared to a car, such as a Ferrari or a Maruti. If we were to conduct a competition between the two cars, running the Ferrari on soda pop and the Maruti on high-quality gasoline, the result would be obvious. Even though Ferrari is having a powerful and better machine, the Ferrari would not be able to function to its full potential, without suitable oil. Just as the body cannot function at its best with poor nutrition. Therefore, it is important to fuel our bodies with good, nutritious food to ensure that we can perform at our best.

Two thousand five hundred years ago Hippocrates 'the father of medicine and a very keen observer, noted that "FAT MEN DIE SUDDENLY" this is still true. In other words, when the waist line increases life line decreases.

You wouldn't head out for a drive without oil in the car's tank, so why start your workout when your personal fuel gauge is approaching empty? Better to workout with some sort of good fuel in your tummy. Just how many calories do you need per day? That depends on a number of things, such as the kind of work you are doing, your age, your body build, and how active you are. A hard working worker may require 5,000 calories a day. To keep going he should need 2,000 calories a day. His wife, who is busy around the house all the day, may need 2,500 calories. But a women office staff may do well with 1,800 calories a day. Below is an approximate sample calorie list of Indian foods.

Calorie-Sheet

Item	Quantity	Caloric value	Item	Quantity	Caloric value
Break fast			**Beverages**		
Egg boiled	1	80	Tea, black, no sugar	1cup	10
Egg fried	1	110	Coffee, black no sugar	1cup	10
Egg omelette	1	120	Tea with milk & sugar	1cup	45
Bread slice with butter	1	90	Coffee, milk & sugar	1cup	45
Chapati	1	60	Milk without sugar	1cup	60
Puri	1	75	Milk with sugar	1cup	75
Paratha	1	150	Horlicks, milk & sugar	1cup	120
Subji	1cup	150	Fresh fruit Juice	1cup	120
Idli	1	100	Aerated soft drinks	1bottle	90
Dosa plain	1	120	Beer	1bottle	200
Dosa masala	1	250	Soda	1bottle	10
Sambhar	1cup	150	Alcohol, neat	1peg, small	75
			Miscellaneous		
Lunch / Dinner			Jam	1tsp	30
Cooked rice, plain	1cup	120	Butter	1tsp	50
Cooked rice, fried	1cup	150	Ghee	1tsp	50
Phulka	1	60	Sugar	1tsp	30
Nan	1	150	Biscuit	1	30
Dal	1cup	150	Fried nuts	1cup	300
Curd	1cup	100	Puddings	1cup	200
Curry, vegetable	1cup	150	Ice-cream	1cup	200
Curry, meat	1cup	175	Milk-shake	1glass	200
Salad	1cup	100	Wafers	1pkt	120
Papad	1	45	Samosa	1	100
Cutlet	1	75	Bhel puri/pani puri	1helping	150
Pickle	1tsp	30	Kabab	1plate	150
Soup, clear	1cup	75	Indian sweet/mithai	1pc	150
Soup, heavy	1cup	150	Fruit	1helping	75

Sample calorie sheet of food items *(https://www.pinterest.com)*

It all depends on how active we are. At 25 years of age, we usually burn up our calories without any difficulty. At 35 the situation begins to change. We are now less active, lie down more often, and perhaps use labour-saving devices to spare us further exertion. This means we must calculate the amount of food according to work we do, and not someone else may be doing.

Are there other conditions that affect a person's weight? Yes, definitely. One may gain weight because of water accumulating in the tissue under the skin. For instance, failing heart may produce marked swellings in the legs and other parts of the body. So will certain kidney diseases. Such people must avoid the excessive use of salt. But this is not the usual reason why most people are overweight. Overeating is more likely to the real problem. How can we change the picture? Two ways, either we must increase the output of work or we must reduce the food intake.

The concept of fuel and energy can be applied to both cars and the human body. Just as a car requires more fuel to travel longer distances at higher speeds, individuals who are more active, work harder, or exercise more frequently will require more calories to sustain their level of activity. Similarly, a car with a more powerful engine will require more fuel to cover the same distance, while individuals with faster metabolisms burn more calories.

During periods of starvation or when calorie intake is reduced, the body will switch to fat metabolism, similar to how hybrid cars switch to the petrol engine when battery power is depleted. This allows the body to continue functioning even when calorie intake is insufficient, ensuring that it can still perform essential functions and maintain overall health.

Maintaining a healthy body requires a balance of diet and exercise, much like how a cycle requires both a front wheel and a back wheel to function properly. To ensure that we are fueling our bodies with nutritious and safe food, it is recommended to keep the kitchen close at hand while keeping the car at a distance to encourage more calorie-burning activities.

Just as a sports car requires high-quality petrol to perform at its best, our bodies also require proper nutrition to function optimally. By fueling our bodies with nutritious food and engaging in regular exercise, we can ensure that our bodies are operating at their highest potential. It is time to reboot, reflect, and dive back into the world of fitness to achieve optimal health and wellness.

It is important not to blindly believe in food advertisements and claims, just as we cannot always trust the mileage claims made by car companies. While a car may be advertised as providing 14 km per litre, we often end up receiving less than that, yet we are still content.

To ensure healthy digestion and bowel movements, it is recommended to consume fiber-rich foods. This can help to reduce the amount of time spent in the bathroom in the morning. Downloading time can be reduced and thus making for a more efficient start to the day.

We can draw a parallel between the process of obtaining a visa and the way we should approach our food choices. Obtaining a visa for an underdeveloped country is often relatively easy because they require foreign money for their survival. However, in developed countries where they have sufficient resources and security measures in place, the visa process is much more stringent. Similarly, we should prioritize the intake of healthy and nutritious food, and avoid treating our stomach as a dumping ground for waste items. Just as a developed country prioritizes its security and safety, we should prioritize our health and well-being by being mindful of the food we consume. We should only "grant a visa" to good, nutritious food that will nourish our bodies and promote optimal health. We can decide the value of our body.

It is imperative that we discard food items that do not contribute to our health and longevity without any hesitation. Our body is considered as the temple of God, and it is our duty to maintain it in optimal shape and working condition. In order to achieve this, we must pay close attention to the types of food we consume, and eliminate those that have a negative impact on our overall well-being. By doing so, we can ensure that our body remains healthy and functional, and we can continue to lead a happy and fulfilling life. It is essential that we prioritize our health above all else, and make conscious decisions about our diet in order to achieve this.

Our body can be likened to coal, in the sense that without oxygen, coal can turn into ash or charcoal. Similarly, our body's 75 trillion cells require water to function properly. Without sufficient water intake, our bodies can become dehydrated, which can have negative effects on our health. Water is an essential component of our body, making up a major part of our body weight. It is often referred to as the internal air conditioner, as it helps regulate body temperature and keeps our organs functioning properly. Therefore, it is important to stay properly hydrated by drinking plenty of water throughout the day, to ensure our bodies are functioning optimally.

Just as we don't wait for our car engine to break down before we change the oil, we shouldn't eat too much junk food that can clog our arteries and damage our heart. Junk food is like a combination of grease and rust that builds up inside the metal pipe that delivers water to your house, and then you need a plumber to fix it. The plumber is like your cardiologist who will have to bypass or remove the affected part and replace it with a new one. A cracked pipe needs to be welded first before it can withstand more pressure. Hot water, which is closer to our body temperature, helps digestion. When we wash a greasy pan, we use hot water that makes the blood vessels dilate. This cleans the inside and allows the blood to flow more easily.

It is said that we eat almost the size of six elephants during our lifetime. However, we can improve our digestion and assimilation by eating smaller, more frequent meals throughout the day. This can also increase our energy levels and reduce lethargy, as well as help reduce body fat. It's interesting to note that marriage advertisements are now changing their focus from fair skin to healthy and glowing skin, emphasizing the importance of overall health and wellness.

Professor Brian Wasnik, author of the amazing book mindless eating, has conducted some extraordinary experiments that show convincingly that when we are distracted during the process of eating, we not only notice what we are eating, we eat substantially more of it. You can probably remember for yourself a time when you were eating popcorn, nuts or crisps while watching a film or a football match. By the time you 'woke up 'and came to your senses, the entire bowl, bag or packet was gone, no matter how hungry you were when you started.

Life is not like a restaurant, where you can eat and then pay, Life is like a food court, where you pay first and then get to eat. A person's health depends on how much care and effort they put in. It's important to remember that nourishment happens through various factors, including air, soil, water, food, and our relationships. Cravings can often be curbed with plain water or social interactions, such as talking to a good friend. Yo-yo dieting can lead to the loss of muscle mass along with fat, and when the weight is regained, it's mostly fat.

Sugary drinks and fast foods provide glucose to the bloodstream quickly, causing the body to store excess energy and leading to a rapid drop in blood sugar levels. This, in turn, triggers hunger pangs shortly after consumption. For instance, a cup of ice cream containing 500 calories can be burned off by an hour of brisk walking or jogging. This highlights how easy it is to consume calories and how challenging it can be to burn them off.

In the fast-paced modern world, it's important to find opportunities to relax and unwind. Celebrations are a common way to do so, and we often indulge in food during these times, whether we're happy or sad. However, it's important to be mindful of our eating habits, even during these festive occasions. One way to do so is to eat smaller portions. For example, while it may be tempting to eat a full meal after drinking a glass of apple juice, it's actually better to eat one whole apple instead. This is because the satiety value of apples is higher than that of apple juice. We tend to take less quantity of meal after the apple compared to juice. By being mindful of our food choices, we can still enjoy celebrations without overindulging and maintain a healthy balance in our lives.

The famous Einstein's equation $E = MC^2$ states that energy cannot be created or destroyed, but can only change forms. This principle applies to our daily lives as well. The energy we consume through food is used by our bodies for physical activity, and any excess energy is stored in the form of fat. To maintain a stable weight, the energy intake from food and the energy expended through physical activity need to be balanced. If there is a surplus of energy intake, the excess energy is stored as fat and can lead to weight gain. Conversely, if there is a deficit of energy intake, the body will use stored fat as energy and result in weight loss.

There is a humorous saying that goes "Green tea can help you lose weight, but only if you climb the mountain and pick the leaves yourself." This highlights the fact that some products marketed as healthy or natural may not be as effective as they claim, and that a more active and natural lifestyle may be the best way to achieve health goals. When it comes to packaged food, it's important to be aware of the ingredients and their nutritional value. However, many ingredients list on packaged foods can be difficult to read and understand, even for experts in the field. Some products may even use vague or misleading terms to describe their ingredients, making it hard for consumers to make informed choices.

It is true that India is known as the yoga capital of the world, but unfortunately, it is also known as the diabetic capital of the world due to the high prevalence of diabetes in the country. When it comes to consuming desserts, it's important to be mindful of portion sizes and to practice moderation. One way to do this is to follow the "three bites rule," where the first bite is a greeting, the second is for enjoyment, and the third is a farewell. This can help satisfy a craving for sweets without overindulging and consuming excess calories. For those with a sweet tooth, it's important to limit the availability of sweets at home. This can be done by not storing excess sweets in the house and instead giving them to friends and relatives. This can help reduce the temptation to overconsume sweets and ultimately lead to the storage of excess fat.

Vitamin D is an essential nutrient required for the proper functioning of the body. However, due to changing lifestyles and increased urbanization, many children are not exposed to enough sunlight, resulting in vitamin D deficiency. This deficiency can lead to weakened bones, muscle weakness, and other health problems. According to child specialist associations, children should be exposed to sunlight for at least 20 minutes every day to maintain adequate levels of vitamin D. Unfortunately, in urban areas, children may not have access to safe outdoor spaces or may spend most of their time indoors, leading to an increased risk of deficiency. Moreover, the problem of vitamin D deficiency is not limited to children alone. The urban Indian population, in general, is also suffering from this issue, with an estimated 80% of people being deficient in this vital nutrient.

Nutrition-TIPS

- *Reduce tummy with neck exercise - The most effective exercise to decrease the tummy is neck exercise. Whenever someone ask you to eat food move your neck to left and right. This means that they don't want any more food, so that you can reduce the calorie consumption.*
- Thank God that air we breathe are calorie free, just as the case for the water we drink. In future there is chance to add odour to the air to make it more refreshing.

- Edited photos can lie, but your body is your ultimate visiting card in today's ambitious, perfectionist world. The only bodily tissue that keeps you looking young, strong and fertile is muscle. Strength training will create an after burn lasting 36-48 hours

- Just as both rain and sunshine are needed to create a rainbow; both joy and sorrow are needed to make life truly beautiful and colourful. We may project the rosy picture around us (especially on social media) but we know where our shoe pinches.

- A myth to be rectified. As long as I exercise it's ok to whatever you want to eat, really think so. Do you think as long as you drive your car it doesn't matter what you put into it, kerosene, petrol, diesel? People always smarter about their cars than their bodies. Exercise is adopting a better lifestyle not an alternative to eating right.

- During purchase and eating, think global and eat local. There is a more chance to freshness and less chance for pesticides in the locally produced items. Do not permit everything to your tummy like a cow. Understand your stomach and accordingly fill it with appropriate items.

- Early to bed and early to rise will make the human healthy, wealthy and wise was the age-old good concept that we were following. Now the food habits are totally changed, dinning out in the night and over consumption of high calorie food is a usual routine for many. Loading at night is the main cause of increased body weight and hypokinetic diseases. Intake of too much carbohydrates and lack of protein and good fats are the main deficiency of our diet.

- Proper nutrition can produce happy hormones like endorphin, oxytocin and serotonin, so that the person can feel young and quite relaxed. This will definitely increase skin glow and beauty.

- Do not shop while hungry-There will be a tendency to purchase more quantity and junk food. Buy smaller plates-plate size also can decide the quantity of intake. When the plate is small and the food is served, we have a feeling of consumed a decent quantity food compared to a big plate.

- Have a food that signals the end of your meal -A small chocolate piece can serve this purpose. Thus, the tummy will get a signal that the food intake has come to the end.

- Supplements are like an insurance policy, but that's not the license to drive the car through the centre of the road. Likewise proper nutritious food is necessary even if you are taking supplements.

- Vegetarian food is more advisable for human digestive system. Vegetarian food can increase the fibre content and can reduce the tiredness. A lion which eats exclusively flesh, sleeps twenty-four hours a day. An orangutan, which eats exclusively plants, sleep six. Vegetable food items are easy to digest and will bring less tiredness to the body. Live body will build from live food. Food that is alive is food with high water content.

- Do not avoid sun, make advantage of it, but too much can cause burn, opens the pores of the skin and escape the toxins. Vitamin D is vital for metabolism and positive mood.

- The dinner must be light for better digestion and sleep. Post sunset digestion slows down. The old usage is very relevant "Breakfast like a king, Lunch like a prince and dinner like a beggar".

- Quick diet produces quick results with quick relapses. As the great philosopher Goethe said "It's not so important where we stand but the direction in which we are moving is important".

- Proper nutrition without proper workouts is like trying to drive a car with a full tank but a flat tire. Many fat reduction advertisements are gimmick that will not burn the fat but will burn a hole in your pocket. Proper diet and exercise are the only way to achieve the goal.

- The three S's - sitting on the floor while eating, switching off gadgets, and eating according to one's senses and hunger cues - can contribute to healthy eating habits. Additionally, policymakers can take steps to increase the availability and accessibility of healthy food choices by introducing a junk food tax and making healthy options more convenient and affordable.

Weight reduction

Dieting is not new to most people who are overweight. They have all tried these many times before. Some are so annoyed at what their friends are saying about them that they will go without food entirely for a short time, only to return again to their former habits of overeating. Going to extremes rarely does any permanent good. The only solution is a completely new pattern of living, such as these simple steps outlined here:

1. Take smaller quantities of food. Continue with a balanced diet. Be sure to include enough fruits vegetables and whole grain in your diet. Eating slowly will help. Stay away from foods that are greasy or high in fat.

2. Be careful about "left-overs" Many housewives put on weight because they hate to see food wasted. Far better to prepare less food and avoid the problem of left overs.

3. Stop nibbling between meals-Train yourself to get along on less food. Soon you will enjoy living on a reduced diet, and you will be surprised at how well you feel.

4. Sensible Exercise taken every day will help to use up those extra calories. The best exercise is walking. Putting those large leg muscles to work will burn up unwanted calories.

5. Avoid rich desserts. All that excess sugar and fat is high in calories but low in food value. Your best "exercise" to push you away from the table while you are still hungry. Stay away from ice cream, pastry, rich cakes and sweets. You can consume these desserts and ice creams, in moderation if you are interested, otherwise, cravings may develop, leading to overindulgence in sweets and worsening the situation beyond the initial state.

6. Regular eating is important. Your meals should be smaller than average, well-prepared and attractively arranged on the table. There is no reason for you not to enjoy your meals, even though you are now taking less food than you once thought you needed.

7. Do not go hungry for long. Eating regularly but sparingly is the best way to lose weight. Long-term starvation can induce a sense of combativeness in the body, making it feel as if a dangerous situation is occurring. As obtaining food may become challenging, similar to during war, the body may start storing more fat for future use, leading to a higher likelihood of overeating. Consequently, the intended goal of achieving sustenance will not be fulfilled, and the opposite effect may ensue.

8. Be sure to have a good breakfast. This will carry you through the day, and you will be less tempted to nibble sweets and snacks between meals.

9. You can eat as much as you want of these foods: green leafy vegetables, fruits that are not sprayed with pesticides and are grown with plenty of fertilizer.

10. However, some individuals may resort to taking diet pills in an attempt to suppress their hunger signals and eat less. They may also sacrifice sleep and experience diuretic effects as a result. Optimal health can be achieved by consuming whole foods as often as possible.

Bringing the weight down to normal will help the heart and every other organ in the body. It takes real will power to lose weight, but it is certainly worthwhile. Once you have reached your ideal weight, make sure that you stay there. You must maintain this new way of life not only for the next month, but for the rest of your days. Once you have accepted this new way of living, you will find yourself enjoying your meals more. Your appetite will be taken with new appreciation of food flavours you never knew before. All this adds up to better health and greater satisfaction in living. Certainly, it pays to control your weight.

Beware of models on the magazines, most of the pictures seen on the cover pages have been digitally altered in order to make the cover striking, so that you will buy the magazine. They are not representative of reality. Never try to copy this unreal image, which make you feel inferior. Rather than constantly compare yourself to something that doesn't exist, it's far better to compare yourself to yourself.

Control-Carvings

Alt -Food Habits

Delete-Stress

Many individuals only begin to control their diet after they have reached a point where they can no longer bear to look at themselves in the mirror due to their negligence and carelessness towards their food intake, or when their clothes no longer fit. This is akin to locking your garage after your car has already been driven away; it's too late, and the damage has been done. The proverbial saying, "A stitch in time saves nine," is very much applicable here.

Our taste preferences can sometimes limit our food choices to unhealthy options. While a single indulgence in high-calorie or junk food may not have significant negative impacts on our health, consistent consumption of such foods can be detrimental to our bodies. It is comparable to how a single pebble cannot shatter a window, but a multitude of pebbles can. Therefore, we should occasionally allow ourselves to deviate from strict calorie counting or healthy eating habits, such as during a party, without worrying about negative consequences. However, constantly subjecting our bodies to unhealthy foods and excessive consumption of bakery items can cause harm and lead to various diseases and health problems. It is important to avoid this kind of consistent abuse of improper diet and prioritize a balanced and healthy diet for our overall well-being.

The quality of our digestion affects not only our physical health, but also our mental well-being. There is a say, that death sits in the bowels, and that the way to a man's heart is through his stomach. Food can be a powerful medicine for our mood, but it can also be a poison. For example, high sugar intake can worsen depression, while a single gut bacterium found in yogurt can reverse the effect of depression. Therefore, we should pay attention to what we eat and how it affects our mind.

Do you know how vitamins and glucose work in your body? Vitamins are not the fuel that gives you energy, but they are the spark that ignites the fuel and keeps your metabolism running. Glucose is like the money you earn every month, while glycogen is like the savings you keep in the bank. You can use your monthly income for your daily expenses, but you need your savings for unexpected emergencies. Similarly, you can use glucose for your immediate energy needs, but you need glycogen for longer periods of activity. However, not all sources of vitamins and glucose are the same. Technology can create artificial wheat in the lab, with all the same chemical components as natural wheat, but it will not grow in the soil. It lacks the life force that makes natural wheat alive and nutritious. The same is true for synthetic vitamins and nutrients. They may look like the real thing, but they are not.

Fruits and Vegetables

Eating a variety of vegetables and fruits is essential for a healthy diet. Different types of vegetables and fruits provide different nutrients that our body needs to function well. By eating plenty of them every day, we can lower our risk of many chronic diseases, such as high blood pressure, heart disease, stroke, cancer, and diabetes. We can also improve our eye health and digestion. Therefore, we should include vegetables and fruits of different colors and textures in our meals and snacks.

Mango, known as the king of fruit, is a tropical fruit that is loved for its sweet taste and juicy flesh. Apart from being delicious, it is also packed with nutrients such as vitamin C, vitamin A, and dietary fiber. These nutrients can help boost the immune system, improve vision health, and aid in digestion. The mango is a fruit that has a special place in Hindu mythology. According to the Vedas, the mango is a heavenly fruit that originated in India. One legend says that when Lord Shiva and Parvathi came down from the Himalayas, they missed eating this delicious fruit. Parvathi, who loved mangoes, asked her husband to create a mango tree by his divine power. Lord Shiva granted her wish and thus the mango tree was born in India.

When it comes to fruits and vegetables, appearance is not everything. In fact, fruits and vegetables that look spotless and flawless may have a higher chance of being adulterated with chemicals or pesticides. On the other hand, locally produced items that have a natural taste and appearance may be more nutritious and safer. Therefore, we should not judge fruits and vegetables by their looks, but by their quality and freshness. Buying from small vendors is a good thing, as it supports local production and provides income to these low-income families.

You can eat whatever you want, just don't eat as much as you want. Variety of nutrients and purchasing power of the people are increasing day by day. But many are ignorant about the nutritional contents the food items and their individual needs. Everyone is unique and the nutritional of needs also differ. Overnutrition makes more people sick than undernutrition. Overweight and obesity are the by-products of over nutrition. The war between overnutrition and undernutrition is widely evident in the society. Rich is becoming richer and poorer is becoming poorer.

Immediately after the workout you have to take some protein, your muscles are in broken state, the protein intake can trigger the recovery process and muscle building. Picture this, your home has got fire and the very place you live is being destroyed. Would you want the fire truck to take the longest route possible to your house. Small amount of dehydration can mean that you have less total blood volume circulating throughout your body-exerting more pressure to heart to pump blood and thus exerting less pressure on arteries. Thus, lowered blood pressure.

If you were to build a new addition to your house and you brought huge pile of bricks to do the job, what would happen? not much. You will need workers to actually take those bricks and build the new addition. Think of the workers as the carbohydrates you eat; they are the ones that make use of the bricks.

Children need to be exposed to some dirt and germs to develop a healthy gut and a strong immune system. That's why we should not be too strict about hygiene and cleanliness with them. Sometimes, we should let them eat a piece of fruit that fell on the floor, or play in a muddy park. This way, they can get more diversity in their microbiota, which are the beneficial bacteria that live in their intestines.

Children should not get everything they want, especially junk food and packaged food. Parents should be firm and say no to their unhealthy requests. A little conflict now will help them later. A good educational institution should focus on the overall development of its students. It should provide a healthy and nutritious canteen or health bar for both students and staff. Junk food items should be avoided and replaced with fruits and nuts that can enhance the well-being of everyone.

In conclusion, nutrition plays a critical role in maintaining optimal health and well-being. The food we consume provides the necessary nutrients that our body needs to function correctly, fight off diseases, and support overall health. Eating a balanced diet that includes a variety of fruits, vegetables, whole grains, lean proteins, and healthy fats is crucial in providing the body with essential vitamins, minerals, and fiber. Moreover, it is essential to limit the consumption of processed foods, high in saturated fats, sugar, and salt, which can increase the risk of chronic diseases such as heart disease, diabetes, and obesity.

Incorporating healthy eating habits into daily life is essential in achieving long-term health benefits. Additionally, staying hydrated is essential for good health as water plays a crucial role in maintaining the body's functions. It's important to remember that nutrition is not a one-size-fits-all solution, and individual needs may vary based on age, sex, lifestyle, and underlying health conditions.

Overall, a healthy and balanced diet, combined with regular physical activity, can help prevent chronic diseases, promote optimal health, and improve overall quality of life. By making small, sustainable changes to our diet and lifestyle, we can work towards achieving optimal health and well-being.

> ***I will never forget your commandments, for you have used them to restore my joy and health.***
>
> **–Bible** (Psalms 119: 93)

3

Workout During Work

"As wealth is essential for the appropriate fulfillment of desire Similarly for the salvation of life, Healthy physique is essential"

–Veda

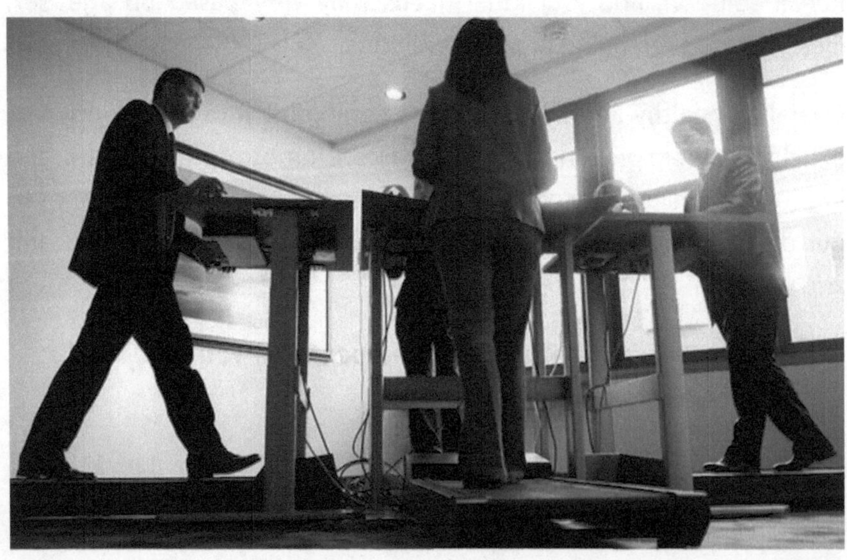

Source: https://www.nytimes.com/2011/12/04/jobs/working-out-inside-the-office.html

One way to promote physical activity in the workplace is to have walking meetings. This is what Salo, a financial staffing firm in Minneapolis, does. They have four treadmill desks in a conference room, where employees can walk and talk at the same time. The desks are height-adjustable and face each other. They also have six more treadmill desks with computers in another room, where employees can walk and work whenever they want. To make things more fun, they also have a Ping-Pong table in the office. Salo's director of operations and administration, Craig Dexheimer, said that walking meetings were a bit strange at first, but now they are normal.

Walking during the day can have positive effects on office workers' mood and performance, according to two studies. One study by the University of Birmingham involved 56 sedentary employees who were asked to walk for 30 minutes at lunchtime, at least three times a week. The researchers measured their stress, enthusiasm, workload and other factors before and after the walks. They found that the walkers had more enthusiasm, relaxation and less nervousness at work than the non-walkers. Another study found that using a treadmill desk can improve memory and attention-to-detail tasks. These findings suggest that walking can benefit both the mental and physical health of office workers.

Exercising during your workday can have many benefits for your productivity and well-being, according to several studies. A Swedish study in 2011 found that more physical activity at work could lead to higher productivity. Another study reported by the Harvard Business Review found that exercising during the day could boost creativity and mental stamina. These studies show that exercising is not only good for your body, but also for your mind and your work performance.

Exercise at desk

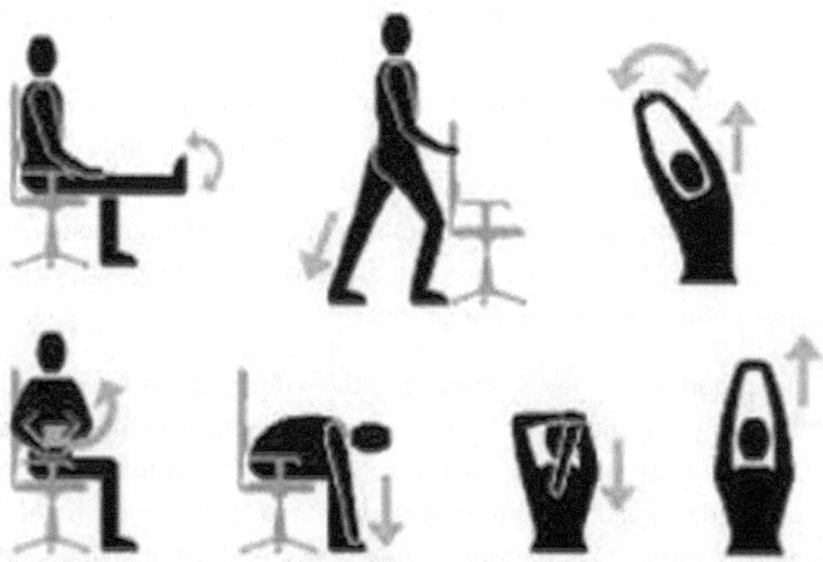

Many people who work at desks suffer from lack of physical activity, which can harm their health. A recent survey showed that this was the most common complaint among desk workers, with more than half of them reporting it. On the other hand, non-desk workers complained mostly about being exhausted from standing all day. This is an ironic contrast between the two types of workers.

Working at a desk all day may seem appealing to some people, but it can have serious side effects on our health. Desk workers often spend too much time indoors, without enough sunlight and fresh air. They also tend to move less, which can lead to weight gain and poor circulation. Moreover, they often adopt hunched-over typing positions, which can cause back pain, neck strain, and eye fatigue. Therefore, working at a desk all day is not as good as it may seem.

Losing weight is a feasible goal that can be achieved through a balanced program of moderate food consumption and daily exercise. However, individuals with desk jobs may face obstacles to their health due to the sedentary nature of their work. In addition to contributing to weight gain, office work can also strain the back, wrists, eyes, and neck, and reduce muscle tone. Stress is another disadvantage of office work that can lead to depression, cardiovascular disease, and low energy levels, among other health issues. A Yale University survey revealed that 29% of workers experience high levels of stress at work. Therefore, it is important for individuals with desk jobs to make conscious efforts to stay active, maintain proper posture, and manage their stress levels to improve their overall health and well-being.

While you shouldn't give up on your home or gym exercise routine, you can certainly supplement it with exercises done at your desk. Here are a few aerobic tricks to try during your next break between tasks:

- One-minute low impact exercises like spot jumping, jumping jacks, back kick, picking up etc. can be performed
- Do a football-like drill of running in place for 60 seconds. Get those knees up! (Beginners, march in place.)
- Simulate jumping rope for a minute: Hop on alternate feet or on both feet at once. An easier version is to simulate the arm motion of turning a rope, while alternately tapping the toes of each leg in front.
- While seated, pump both arms over your head for 30 seconds, and then rapidly tap your feet on the floor, football-drill style, for 30 seconds. Repeat 3-5 times.
- If you can step into a vacant office or conference room, shadow box for a minute or two. Or just walk around the room as fast as you can. Or do walk-lunges in your office or a vacant room.
- No conference rooms? Take to the stairs, two at a time if you need a harder workout! Do this 5-7 times a day.

If you want to stay healthy despite working long hours, you need to exercise. But how can you fit it into your busy schedule? You can try some workplace workouts that don't take much time or space. You can use your breaks, your desk, or your chair to do some simple exercises that will keep you fit. Here are some examples of exercises you can do without anyone noticing.

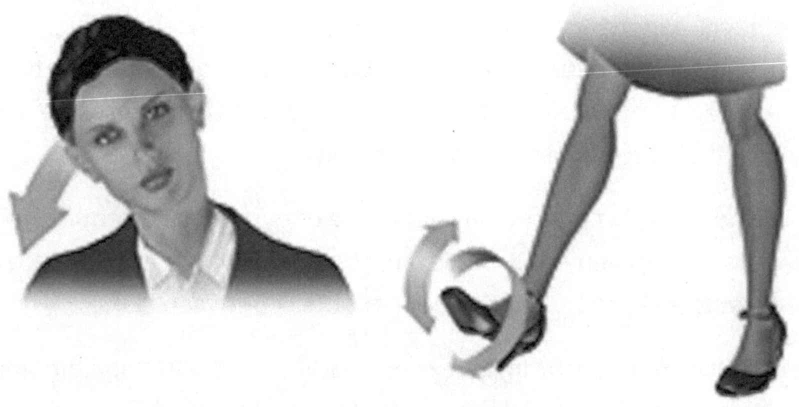

Source-https://health.howstuffworks.com/wellness/diet-fitness/exercise-at-work/10-office-exercises-you-can-do-secretly.htm

For a full-body joint flexion exercise, start by flexing all joints from the head to toe and repeating the movement ten times for each joint to help improve overall flexibility and mobility.

- Slowly tilt your head towards one shoulder, hold the position for ten seconds, and then alternate sides by tilting your head towards the other shoulder. Then perform the semi rotation of the neck in forward and backward direction.
- Perform a circular motion by rolling both shoulders forward and backward
- Bend your elbow joint by flexing your arm and then straightening it out again,
- Rotate your wrist joint in a clockwise direction, and then repeat the same motion in an anticlockwise direction, trying to draw a big circle with your wrist.

- To increase hip mobility, try rotating your hip joint in a clockwise and counterclockwise direction by drawing big circles with your hip

- To perform knee flexion and extension exercises, start by sitting in a position where your thighs are parallel to the ground and then stand up, repeating the motion to help strengthen the muscles around your knees.

- To improve ankle mobility, try rotating your ankle joint in a clockwise and counterclockwise direction by making circular motions with your foot.

All the above given exercises can be completed within five minutes. After mobilizing the joints, if time permits, stretching the muscles can also be done from the office or during the next break. There are many YouTube videos available on the internet regarding this topic. Internet browsing is a good method to improve our fitness knowledge, but be careful when implementing new exercises into your training plan, because not all videos are prepared by competent professionals.

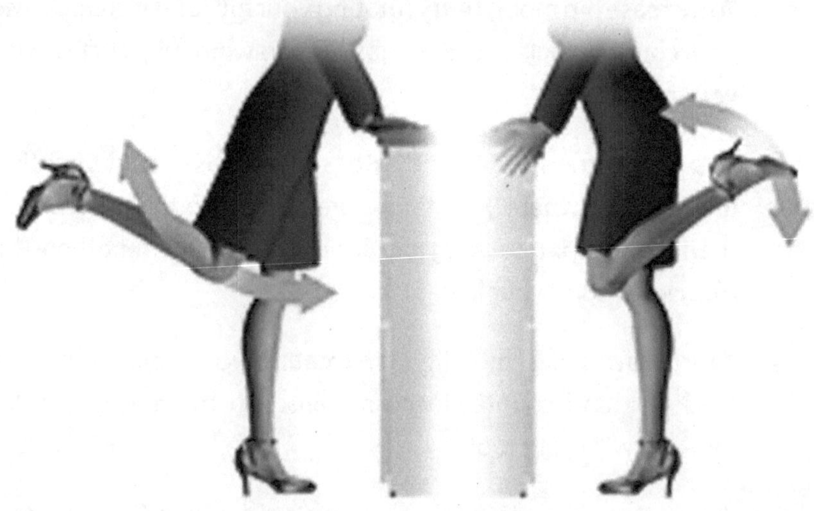

Leg lifts and swings

Make use of your time spent watching copies spew out of the copy machine, you can try incorporating some leg toning and strengthening exercises. For example, you can do squats or lunges while waiting for the copies to finish. Another exercise you can try is calf raises, which involve standing on your tiptoes and lowering your heels back down to the ground.

With leg lifts and swings you use the muscles in the leg you are moving and also use the weight of your body to strengthen the leg you are standing on for support. It's best to hold onto the copy machine for balance. If you hear someone approaching, you can quickly stop.

- Lift one leg to the back or side, keeping it straight.
- Slowly lower it.
- Change sides.
- In the same position, bend your right knee.

- Swing leg forward and back for 30 seconds.
- Repeat with left leg.
- Glute kicks and calf raises will stretch out your hamstrings and calves.
- Stand with one leg straight.
- Try to kick your buttocks with the heel of your other leg.
- Repeat ten times with each leg.
- Next, raise your heels off the floor.
- Slowly lower them.
- Repeat ten times.

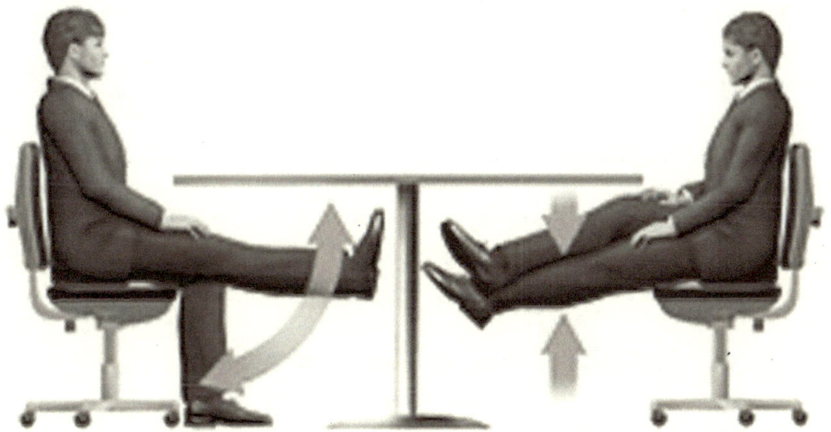

Leg toners

How to act- Your co-workers will see you intently reading the report from yesterday's meeting, but they won't see you strengthening your abs and relieving your tired leg muscles. Start with feet flat on floor.

- Sit tall at your desk.

- Hold your abdominal muscles tight.
- Extend one leg until it is level with your hip.
- Hold for ten seconds.
- Slowly lower leg.
- Repeat 15 times.
- Change legs.

Chair squats are an effective body-strengthening exercise. Sneak a few in every time you get up from your chair and sit back down.

- Stand tall.
- Keep back straight.
- Lower to one inch of chair, pretending you are sitting down.
- Hold for ten seconds.
- Lift back up to standing position.
- You don't need a resistance band to get great leg toning.
- With legs straight, cross one on top of the other.
- Raise them off the floor.
- Press top leg down and resist with bottom leg.
- Do until muscles are tired.
- Repeat with opposite legs top and bottom.
- To keep your projects and your body moving, visit colleagues rather than e-mailing them.

Drink a lot of water. Research suggests that drinking water can aid in your weight loss efforts plus, the more trips to the restroom, the more calories you'll burn. To increase the calorie count, visit a restroom further away from your desk. You might also run into some new people along the way.

Always walk fast without running. It'll get your heart beating faster and make it look like you have somewhere important to be.

Take the stairs whenever possible instead of elevator. For a better workout, take the steps two at a time.

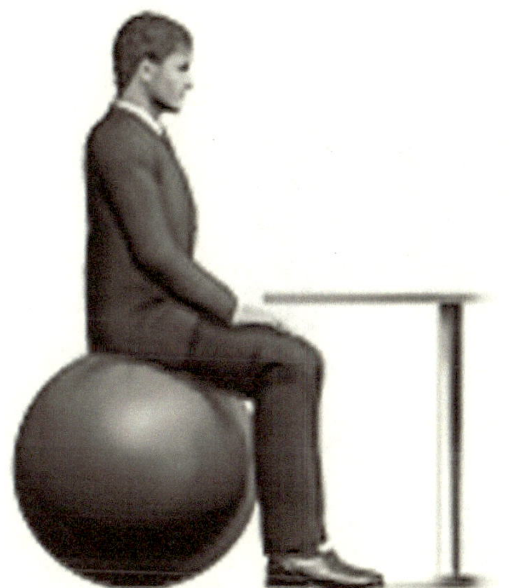

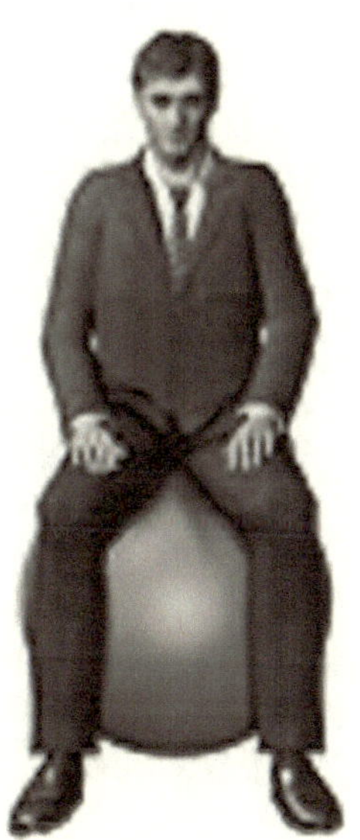

Exercise ball

If you want to tone and strengthen your abdominal muscles throughout the day, sometimes, consider replacing your office chair with an exercise ball. Sitting on an exercise ball forces you to engage your abs to maintain proper balance and posture. This can help improve your core strength, reduce lower back pain and even enhance your concentration. However, it's important to gradually build up your tolerance to sitting on an exercise ball and to maintain proper posture to prevent injury.

- Sit on the ball and find your balance.
- Pull your navel in.
- Pull your shoulders back (no slouching).
- Place feet hip width apart.

Sitting on an exercise ball isn't easy. You might want to try it at home first to see how long you can last.

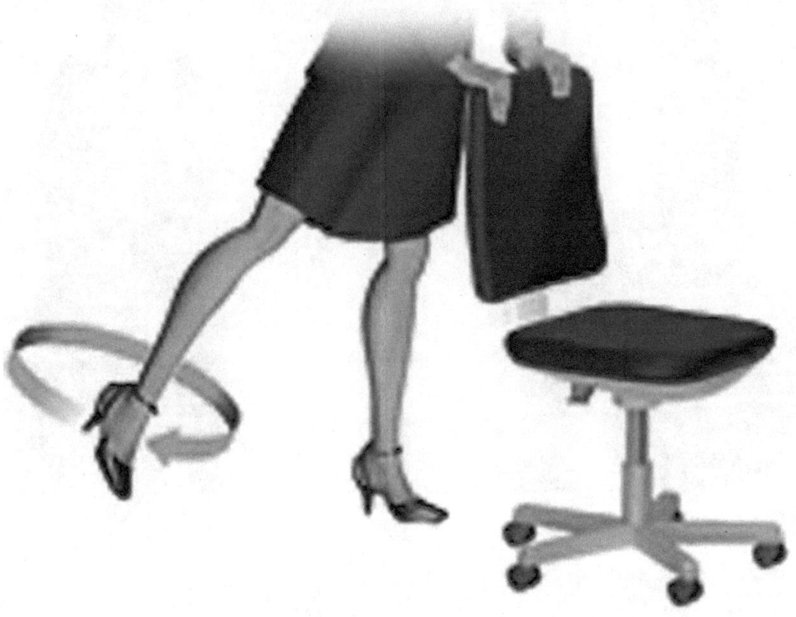

Arabesque

- While you're focused on helping your company increase its bottom line, don't forget to take care of your own health and well-being. Incorporating exercises to tighten and strengthen your gluteus muscles can not only help you achieve a more toned and defined backside, but can also help alleviate back pain. Some exercises you can try include squats, lunges, glute bridges, and fire hydrants. Additionally, incorporating some stretching exercises like the seated spinal twist or the standing hamstring stretch can help relieve tension in your lower back. Remember to start with proper form and gradually increase the intensity and frequency of your exercises for best results.

- Lift one glute up and almost off the chair.
- Perform in a side-to-side rocking motion for 30 seconds.
- Next, squeeze your gluteus muscles.
- Hold for ten seconds.
- Release.

Arabesque circle exercises, originally designed for dancers, can be an effective way to tone your glutes and hamstrings while you're on the phone. To perform this exercise, stand facing your desk with one hand on the desk for support. Lift one leg behind you and draw a small circle with your foot, keeping your leg straight. Repeat the motion several times before switching to the other leg. This exercise is best performed in a private office to avoid distraction or embarrassment

- Stand with your feet shoulder-width apart.
- Shift weight to left leg.
- Lift right leg behind you.
- Hold on to your desk or chair for balance.
- Slowly circle your left leg clockwise 25 times and counter-clockwise 25 times.
- Switch legs.

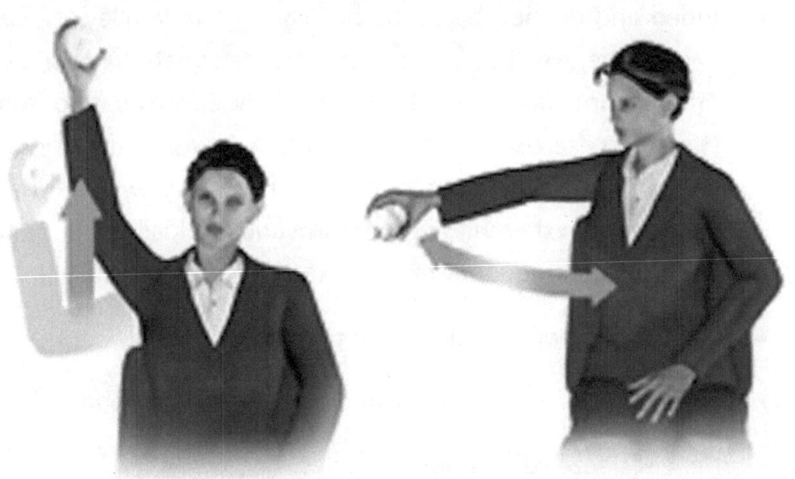

Front raises and twists

You don't need to invest in expensive weights to tone and strengthen your arms. Instead, try using a full water bottle or a bottle filled with water as a substitute for a dumbbell. If someone interrupts you, you can simply take a drink and continue your workout later. Start with bicep curls by holding the water bottle in your hand and bending your elbow to lift the bottle towards your shoulder. Slowly lower the bottle back down and repeat for several reps. Another option for a makeshift dumbbell is using a bottle filled with sand, which can also be used for toning and strengthening exercises.

- Sit tall with abs pulled in
- Hold water bottle in right hand and curl it up towards your shoulder.
- Repeat 15 times.
- Change arms.
- You can also use your water bottle to do front arm raises and overhead presses.

- Hold water bottle in right hand.
- Bend elbow.
- Extend arm overhead.
- Repeat other side.
- Water bottle twists are a great way to work your waistline.
- Hold water bottle at chest level.
- Twist to the right as far as you can.
- Twist back to center.
- Twist to the left.
- Repeat 10 times.

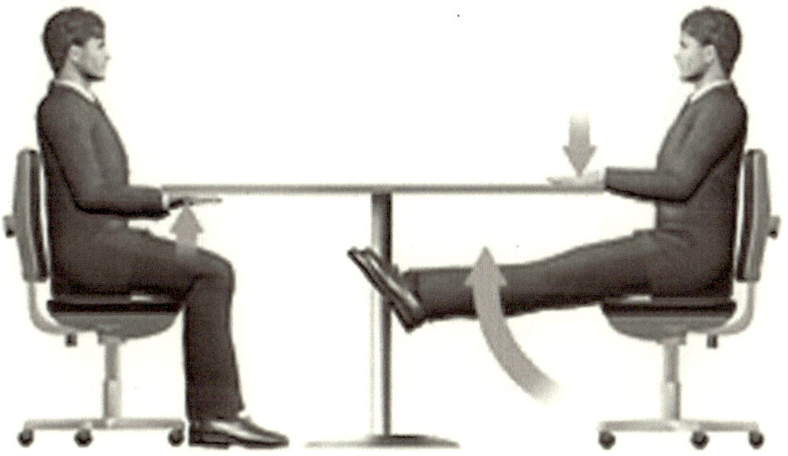

Leg lifts

How to act - Just because you are sitting still during meetings, doesn't mean you can't be exercising. You can use the conference room table to do a variety of toning and strengthening exercises.

- First try to lift the table.

- Put your hand under the table.
- Press up against the table.
- Continue until your muscles are tired.
- Do this one hand at a time or both together. Next, push the table into the floor.
- Put hand on table, palm down.
- Press down as strongly as you can.
- Stop when your muscles are tired.
- You can do this one hand at a time or both together if it looks more natural.
- Using a shoulder shrug when answering, "I don't know" allows you to work in this exercise.
- Raise the top of your shoulders toward ears.
- Hold for three to five seconds.
- Relax.
- You'll appear attentive, while exercising your whole body with this move.
- Sit on the edge of chair.
- Press down on table with both hands.
- At same time lift legs as high as you can.

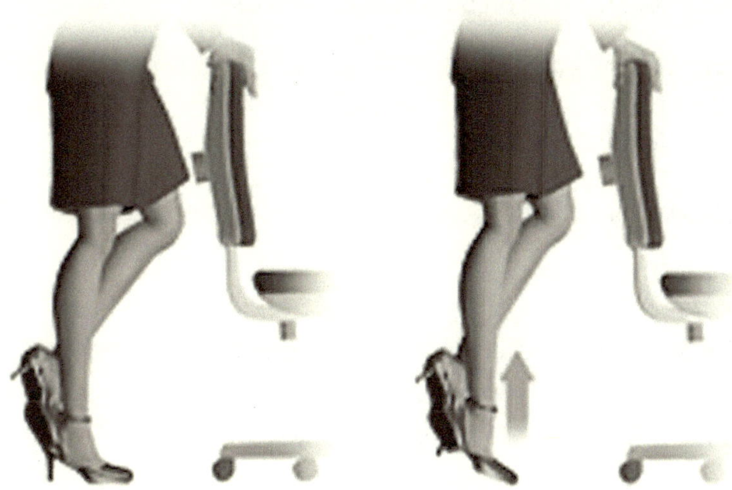

Calf raises

Isometric exercises, also known as static strength training, can be performed without any visible joint movement, making them a great option for exercises that can be done unnoticed. For those who spend extended periods on the computer, hand squeezes can help alleviate tension in the fingers, and can be done with or without a stress ball.

- Make a fist.
- Squeeze.
- Hold and release.
- Stretch fingers.
- Repeat ten times
- Strengthen your calves and ankles while you read, listen to a web cast or talk on the phone.
- Stand and hold onto your chair.

- Rest your left foot on back of your right calf.
- Raise up on your toes.
- Hold for 20-30 seconds.
- Repeat three times.
- Change legs.

Kegel exercises are an effective way to strengthen your pelvic floor muscles and prevent or control urinary incontinence. These exercises can be done discreetly while performing any routine task.

- Contract your pelvic floor muscles.
- Hold for five seconds.
- Relax.
- Repeat five times, three times a day.

You can use this squeeze, hold and release technique to strengthen just about any muscle.

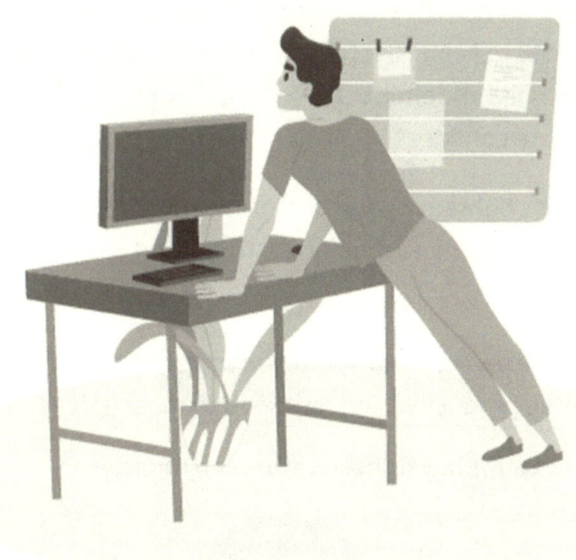

Desk Plank

- Place your hands shoulder-width apart on the edge of your desk.
- Walk your feet back, shifting your weight forward until your arms are straight and your body is in a straight line from shoulders to feet.
- To do a plank, keep your core and glutes tight while holding the position for 30 seconds.

Sometimes the best way to burn calories isn't by exercising at all. Following are a few non-exercise ways to shed some weight.

- Stand whenever you can. You'll burn more calories than sitting, as many as 50 more an hour for a 70kg person
- Fidgeting can burn an extra calorie. Rapidly tapping your feet, talking with your hands, and chewing gum, all count.

Good posture is an effective core strengthening measure. It requires you to use muscles to keep your tummy tight and your back straight. Do it continually to build abdominal strength, alleviate lower back pain and help you feel more confident.

Laugh often. It tightens your stomach muscles, exercises your diaphragm, works your heart, relieves stress and gives you a better outlook on life.

By making exercise part of your everyday work routine, you'll be healthier, happier and more productive. But let's keep that our little secret.

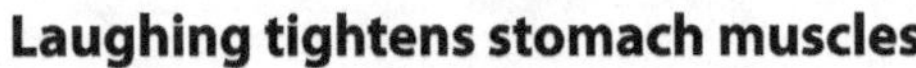

Laughing tightens stomach muscles

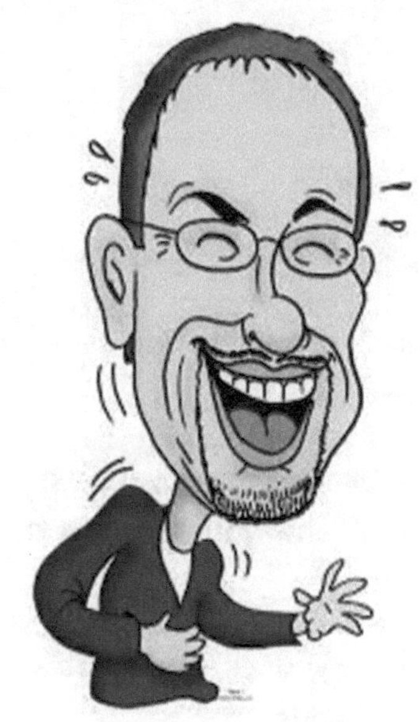

Additional Tips to become fit in the office

- Take short exercise breaks every 30-60 minutes.
- Walk around the office or building during breaks.
- Use resistance bands or hand weights at your desk.

- Practice desk pushups for upper body strength
- Try wall sits to build leg strength.
- Take a brisk walk during lunch or break time.
- Do jumping jacks for a quick cardio burst.
- Take a break to do some yoga poses.
- Do triceps dips on the edge of your desk or chair.
- Use a foam roller to stretch your muscles.
- Take a 5-minute dance break to get your heart pumping.
- Use a stability ball for exercises like crunches and bridges.
- Do high knees or butt kicks for a quick cardio burst.
- Take a few minutes to meditate and breathe deeply.
- Use a resistance band to do bicep curls or overhead presses.
- Use a balance board to engage your core and improve balance.
- Use a medicine ball for exercises like Russian twists and wall throws.
- Use ankle weights for leg exercises.
- Use a pull-up bar to build upper body strength.
- Do side planks for core and oblique strength.
- Use a kettlebell for exercises like swings and squats.

To keep the body in good health is a duty... otherwise we shall not be able to keep our mind strong and clear.

–Buddha

4

Myths About Fitness

"My child I want is muscles of iron and nerves of steel, inside which dwells the mind of the same material as that of which the thunderbolt is made"

–Swami Vivekananda

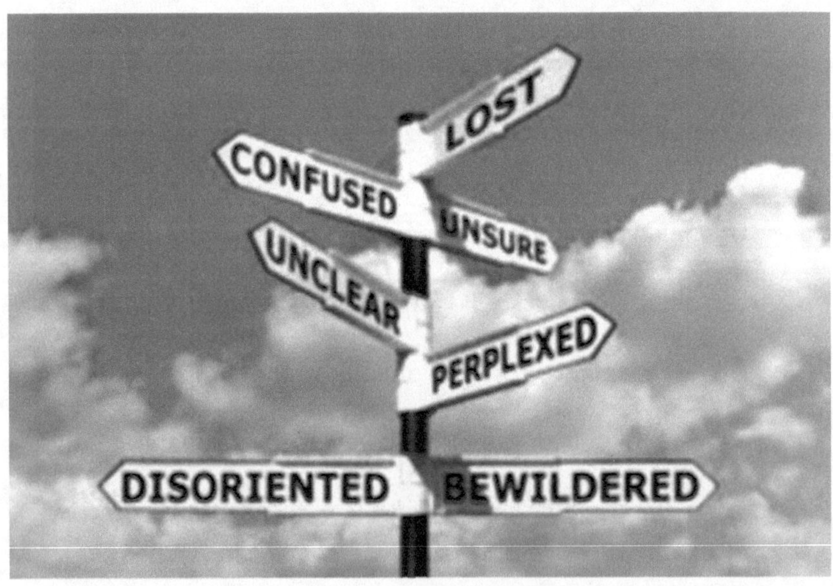

Source: https://www.pinterest.com/pin/44332377559549043/

1) **Is six- pack is the measure of fitness?**

Having a muscular body does not necessarily mean that a person is physically fit, as bodybuilders often focus solely on isolating specific muscles for aesthetic purposes while neglecting other important exercises like stretching and cardiovascular activities. Achieving complete fitness requires a well-rounded workout routine that includes exercises for flexibility, endurance, speed, coordination, and strength. The nature of our bodies is unchangeable, just like the tides of the ocean, and there are no quick fixes or targeted fat reduction techniques in fitness journeys. Consistency is more important than intensity, and making revolutionary decisions based on external stimuli like watching a movie or witnessing someone win an international medal may not lead to lasting changes. To achieve good fitness, slow and methodical progress is necessary, as too much focus on crunches for a six-pack can lead to injuries in the abdomen and back. It's essential to mix up activities to achieve perfect fitness because no one event can activate all 600+ skeletal muscles in the human body.

2) **Running on treadmill is same as running on outside?**

Running on a treadmill is an assisted activity, as the belt or surface moves beneath your feet with minimal effort required. This means fewer muscles are activated in your body compared to outdoor activities. Instead of relying on a treadmill, consider heading outside for a brisk walk or run, particularly when the weather is pleasant. Not only does being outside allow you to enjoy the benefits of nature as a stress-relieving agent, but it also provides opportunities for socialization. Remember, any activity is better than none, so even a short outdoor walk can be beneficial for your physical and mental health.

3) What is the right running Technique?

In the past, people often ran barefoot or with minimal footwear due to the unavailability of cushioned shoes. Running barefoot can help you find your natural running movement, landing on the midfoot and front part of your foot instead of your heel, which is the correct technique. It's also important to keep the upper body and facial muscles relaxed and to hold your palms loosely cupped with the elbow joint at a 80-90 degree angle. Avoid crossing your arms over the midline of your body, and focus on using your shoulder rather than elbow joint for arm movements. Unnecessary movements during running can lead to energy wastage and injury. Developing strength and flexibility through running ABC exercises can improve your coordination and movement efficiency.

4) Whether Shoe is compulsory for walking or running?

Walking or running barefoot on grass and sand can be very beneficial for the body. The nerve endings on the soles of our feet get stimulated, resulting in overall rejuvenation. While shoes are necessary for proper support and safety during activity, the occasional exposure of feet to natural surfaces can provide maximum benefits.

When purchasing athletic shoes, there are several fitting facts to consider:

- Purchase shoes from a specialty store where staff can assist with fitting and offer advice on the appropriate type of shoe for your sport.
- Buy shoes in the evening when feet are at their largest and wear the same type of sock you would wear during your activity.

- Ensure that you can freely wiggle all of your toes while wearing the shoes and that they are immediately comfortable with no break-in period.
- Walk or run a few steps to ensure comfort and a firm grip on the heel.
- If you participate in a sport three or more times a week, it is recommended to have a sport-specific shoe.
- There are various types of athletic shoes with differences in design, material, and weight, developed to protect the areas of the feet that encounter the most stress during a particular athletic activity.

5) Is walking or jogging on concrete bad for the knees?

The surface you run on can have an impact on your joints, but it's not the only factor. Even if you run on a soft track, if your technique is wrong, you can still damage your knees. The right technique involves using your muscles as shock absorbers to minimize impact on your joints. Running on hard surfaces like pavement can stress your bones, but giving your muscles sufficient rest between runs and strengthening and stretching them can help prevent injury. While soft surfaces like grass and sand are more joint-friendly, Tar roads and interlock areas are considered hard surfaces.

6) Doing excessive crunches or working out on abs machines help me flatten my stomach?

Simply doing crunches alone will not reduce a pot belly, and may even lead to injury if other muscle groups are not exercised properly. In order to burn excess calories, it's important to engage in cardio exercises such as walking, jogging, swimming, dancing, skipping, or climbing. Over-exercising one particular muscle group can cause an imbalance and lead to injury. It's not possible to target fat reduction in a specific area of the body, and abdominal muscles will only become visible once excess fat in that area is reduced. A long-term plan involving proper diet and exercise is necessary to achieve desired results.

7) What is more important for good health: Aerobic fitness or muscular fitness?

Both aerobic and muscular fitness are important components of overall fitness. In the past, there was more emphasis on aerobic fitness, but now we recognize the importance of muscular fitness as well. Aerobic fitness is crucial for preventing cardiovascular disease and some types of cancer, while muscular fitness helps build strong muscles and bones, which can prevent osteoporosis and reduce the risk of musculoskeletal injuries like low back pain. Focusing on one aspect of fitness can improve the other, so it's important to identify weak areas and give them extra attention in your fitness plan. Fitness is a combination of endurance, strength, speed, flexibility, and coordination. For those over thirty strength and Flexibility are especially important factors to focus on.

8) Should I do aerobic exercise or strength training first?

When it comes to the order of aerobic exercise and strength training, it's best to allow for recovery time in between. However, if you don't have that luxury, the order should depend on your fitness goals and preferences. If you want to focus on strength development, it's best to lift weights first since you'll be less fatigued and have a more productive workout. But if you want to improve your cardio respiratory system or enhance calorie expenditure for weight loss, it's better to do aerobic exercise first. This is because heavy lower body lifting can make it difficult to maintain a good cardio workout afterward. Ultimately, it's important to evaluate your goals and select the training order accordingly. Both forms of exercise have their benefits, including increased energy and a more toned appearance. However, it's important to note that while strength training can convert fat to muscle, it won't necessarily reduce overall body weight as muscle tissue is heavier than fat tissue.

9) What is the best fitness activity?

Overall fitness cannot be achieved through a single physical activity, sport, or exercise. Most people tend to stick to one mode of exercise, such as walking, swimming, or jogging. While these activities can contribute to cardio respiratory development, their contribution to other fitness components can vary. To achieve total fitness, it's important to supplement aerobic activities with strength and flexibility programs. Cross-training, or selecting different activities for fitness development and maintenance (such as jogging, water aerobics, or spinning), can add variety and enjoyment to your workout routine while also reducing the risk of injuries from overuse. Just like with our food choices, variety in activities can contribute more to our fitness journey. It's important to have the will and determination to become fit, and even small spaces such as an office room, bedroom, railway station, or airport can become destinations for fitness for those who are committed to their goal.

10) Will exercise help me feel better?

Exercise can indeed help improve one's mood and mental well-being, as evidenced by various studies. Regular exercise can improve self-esteem, confidence, and relieve stress and depression. Exercise can also produce positive hormones in the body while neutralizing the stress hormone cortisol. A lifetime of physical activity is just as important for mental wellness as it is for physical health. Even if you have time constraints, doing some deep breathing and stretching while lying down on the floor can make a significant difference in your mood. This is because lying down allows for better oxygenated blood supply to the brain, unlike sitting or standing positions where gravity pull is towards the lower extremities and less oxygenated blood reaches the brain.

11) Should I exercise when I have a cold or the flu?

When it comes to exercising while sick, it's important to be sensible and listen to your body. If you're experiencing a runny nose, sneezing, or a scratchy throat, it's usually safe to continue with exercise. However, if you have a fever, achy muscles, vomiting, diarrhea, or a persistent cough, it's best to avoid exercise. After recovering from an illness, it's important to ease back into your exercise routine gradually, rather than returning to your pre-illness intensity and duration right away.

12) How fast does a person lose the benefits of exercise after stopping an exercise program?

The rate at which the benefits of exercise are lost depends on the fitness component and the individual's level of fitness. Inactivity can quickly reverse four weeks of aerobic training in just two weeks. However, individuals who have been exercising regularly for months or years may not be affected as much as those who have only exercised for a few weeks. Within two to three days of inactivity, the cardio respiratory system begins to lose some of its capacity. Flexibility can be maintained with two or three stretching sessions per week, and strength can be maintained with just one maximal training session per week. It's important to maintain a regular fitness program even during travel and vacation periods. Before leaving home, plan ahead and examine your options. Many hotels have in-house fitness facilities, although the equipment may be limited. Frequent travelers can benefit from joining a nationally franchised health club or a YMCA. Walking, jogging, and rope jumping are excellent alternatives for exercise on the road. When venturing out in a new city, ask for safe places to jog, such as nearby parks or a high school track, to avoid traffic and stop lights.

13) What type of clothing should I wear when I exercise?

When exercising, the type of clothing you wear is important for comfort and allowing free movement. Clothing should be selected based on the expected air temperature, humidity, and exercise intensity. Avoid tight clothes made of nylon or rubberized materials that interfere with the body's cooling mechanism or obstruct normal blood flow. Fabrics made from polypropylene, Capilene, Thermax, and synthetics are best as they wick moisture away from the skin and enhance evaporation. When exercising in the heat, avoid the hottest time of the day and surfaces that absorb heat. Minimal lightweight, light-colored, loose-fitting, and absorbent clothing is necessary for maximal evaporation. A straw hat can be worn to protect the eyes and head from the sun. Proper footwear is also vital for preventing lower limb injuries. Shoes should be specific to your activity, body type, tendency towards pronation or supination, and exercise surfaces. Good stability, motion control, and a comfortable fit are important features to look for. Shoes with nylon or mesh uppers are best for breathability. It's best to purchase shoes in the afternoon when the feet have expanded, and salespeople at reputable athletic shoe stores can assist in finding the right shoe.

14) What time of the day is best for exercise?

Exercising can be done at any time of the day, except for about two hours following a large meal or during the noon and early afternoon hours on hot and humid days. Many individuals prefer exercising in the morning as it gives them a boost to start their day and minimizes the likelihood of other activities interfering with their exercise regimen. For weight control reasons, some people opt for exercising during lunch hour as it can lead to a smaller lunch, reducing daily caloric intake. People with high levels of stress tend to exercise in the evening as it helps them relax. However, if time permits, morning is the best time for exercise because of the less polluted air and to avoid negative thoughts creeping in the mind.

15) How long should a person wait after a meal before engaging in strenuous physical exercise?

The timing of exercise after eating depends on the amount of food consumed. Generally, it is recommended to wait about 2 hours after a regular meal before engaging in strenuous physical activity. However, light physical activity such as a walk is acceptable immediately after the meal. It is advised to consume small but frequent meals to aid digestion and assimilation. After a light meal, exercise will not harm the body. Heavy meals cause blood to accumulate in the stomach for digestion, leading to feelings of sleepiness and reduced oxygenation to the brain. Engaging in strenuous activity after a heavy meal may interfere with digestion due to the high demand for oxygenated blood in the muscles.

16) How should acute sports injuries be treated?

Prevention is always the best treatment. If an activity causes discomfort or chronic irritation, the cause should be treated by decreasing intensity, switching activities, substituting equipment, or upgrading clothing. In cases of acute injury, rest, cold application, compression or splinting, and elevation of the affected body part should be used, which is commonly known as RICE: Rest, Ice, Compression, Elevation. Cold should be applied three to five times a day for 15 to 20 minutes at a time during the first 36 to 48 hours, using an ice bag, submerging the injured area in cold water, or applying ice massage. An elastic bandage or wrap can be used for compression. Elevating the body part helps to decrease blood flow to it and reduce swelling. After the first 36 to 48 hours, heat can be used if there is no further swelling or inflammation. Seeking medical evaluation is important if there are doubts regarding the nature or seriousness of the injury, or if there are obvious deformities. Splinting, cold application, and medical attention are necessary in cases of fractures, dislocations, or partial dislocations. Resetting these conditions by oneself is not recommended, as it can cause further damage to muscles, ligaments, and nerves. Immediate rubbing after an injury is not recommended, as it can cause vasodilation and more blood flow to the injured area, resulting in increased inflammation. The application of ice causes vasoconstriction, which reduces blood flow to the injured area and inflammation.

17) What causes muscle soreness and stiffness?

Muscle soreness and stiffness are common experiences for individuals who (a) start a new exercise program or return to exercise after a prolonged break, (b) exercise beyond their usual intensity or duration, or (c) engage in eccentric training. The soreness that occurs within a few hours after exercise is due to the accumulation of chemical waste products that cause general fatigue in the worked muscles. Delayed-onset muscle soreness (DOMS), which occurs several hours after exercise and can last for two to four days, may be caused by microtears in muscle tissue, muscle spasms that increase fluid retention and stimulate pain receptors, and overstretching or tearing of connective tissue around muscles and joints.

There are two types of muscle contractions involved in movement: concentric and eccentric. During a concentric contraction, the muscle shortens as it generates tension. During an eccentric contraction, the muscle fibers lengthen while generating tension. For example, when performing a bicep curl, the elbow flexor muscles (biceps, brachioradialis, and brachialis) shorten during the upward motion (concentric contraction) and lengthen during the downward motion (eccentric contraction). When running, the leg muscles contract eccentrically as they absorb the body weight upon landing, followed by a concentric contraction as the leg pushes off the ground to move forward. Cycling, however, requires only concentric contractions of the leg muscles as the quadriceps contract while pushing down on the pedal and the hamstrings contract during the upward motion when using toe clips.

18) What are the recommended guidelines for fluid replacement during prolonged aerobic exercise?

Fluid replacement is crucial during prolonged aerobic exercise to maintain normal circulation and sweating. The primary goal is to prevent heat disorders by replacing water. Drinking 200-250ml of water every 15-20 minutes is recommended to prevent dehydration. Commercial fluid-replacement solutions with 6-8% glucose is ideal for fluid absorption and performance. For exercise lasting less than an hour, water is sufficient to replace fluid loss, but sports drinks are recommended for strenuous exercise over an hour. Choose a sports drink based on personal preference and try different drinks with 6-8% glucose concentration to determine tolerance and taste. Glucose becomes available to muscles after about 30 minutes, and drinks with high fructose or glucose concentrations above 8% can slow water absorption during exercise in heat. Soft drinks with 10-12% glucose is not recommended for proper rehydration. For long-distance events, consume 30-60 grams of carbohydrates (120-240 calories) every hour, ideally by drinking 250 ml of a 6-8% carbohydrate sports drink every 15 minutes.

19) What is more important for weight loss: a negative caloric balance (diet) or increasing physical activity?

The key to losing body weight is to balance calorie intake with calorie expenditure through physical activity and dieting. Dieting determines the calorie intake, while physical activity determines the calorie expenditure. Combining physical activity with dieting leads to accelerated weight loss, and results in more effective changes in body composition, with a greater loss of body fat and preservation of lean body tissue. However, to maintain weight loss, sustained daily physical activity or exercise for 60 to 90 minutes is necessary in most cases.

20) Are some diets plans more effective than others?

Diet plans are commonly used for weight reduction, particularly in cases of overeating and consumption of unhealthy junk food that led to obesity. Creating a negative caloric balance is essential to lose weight, which means that one consumes fewer calories than the body requires to maintain its current weight. Weight loss occurs when the energy expended exceeds the energy intake. There are various popular diets that differ in food choices. Restricting food choices can reduce the risk of overeating, leading to a lower caloric intake, and thus more weight loss. However, it is important to maintain a balanced diet during weight loss, ensuring a variety of nutrients. Health experts recommend a minimum of 1,500 calories per day to sustain good health, emphasizing the consumption of grains, fruits, vegetables, and small amounts of low-fat animal products or fish.

21) Are there specific nutrient requirements for optimal development and recovery following exercise?

In addition to carbohydrates and protein, it's also important to stay hydrated during and after exercise. Water is usually sufficient for activities lasting less than an hour, but for longer activities or activities in hot weather, a sports drink with electrolytes can be beneficial. It's also important to remember that individual needs may vary based on factors such as age, weight, and intensity of exercise. Consulting a healthcare professional or registered dietitian can help determine the best nutrition plan for individual needs and goals.

22) What is the relationship between aging and physical work capacity?

In addition to the physical and psychological benefits, fitness programs for older adults also have social benefits. Older adults who participate in fitness programs have the opportunity to interact with peers and develop new social connections, which can lead to improved social support and an increased sense of well-being. Many fitness programs for older adults are designed to be enjoyable and include group activities, such as dancing or group exercise classes, which can make exercise more enjoyable and increase adherence to the program. It is important for older adults to consult with their healthcare provider before starting any new exercise program and to start at a level that is appropriate for their current fitness level and health status. As individuals progress in their fitness program, they can gradually increase the intensity and duration of their workouts.

23) Do older adults respond to physical training?

Research has demonstrated that older adults can improve their functional fitness and contribute to healthy aging through fitness programs. These programs should aim to develop cardio respiratory endurance, muscular strength and endurance, muscular flexibility, agility and balance, and motor coordination. Systematic physical activity throughout life helps maintain a higher level of functional capacity and prevent declines in later years. Cardio respiratory endurance training helps decrease the risk for disease, improve health status, and increase life expectancy. Strength training helps decrease the rate of strength and muscle mass loss commonly associated with aging, and also preserves cognitive function, reduces symptoms and behaviors related to depression, and improves self-confidence and self-esteem.

Older adults who increase their physical activity experience significant changes in cardio respiratory endurance, strength, and flexibility. The extent of the changes depends on their initial fitness level and the types of activities they select for their training. Improvements in maximal oxygen uptake in older adults are similar to those of younger people, although older people seem to require a longer training period to achieve these changes. The rate of decline in maximal oxygen uptake is slower in people who maintain a lifetime aerobic exercise program. Blood pressure, heart rate, and body weight are also better in the exercising group.

Muscle strength declines by 10 percent to 20 percent between the ages of 20 and 50, but between ages 50 and 70 it drops by another 25 percent to 30 percent. However, frail adults in their 80s or 90s can double or triple their strength in just a few months through strength training. The amount of muscle hypertrophy achieved decreases with age, but strength gains close to 200 percent have been found in previously inactive adults older than 90. Regular strength training also improves balance, gait, speed, functional independence, morale, depression symptoms, and energy intake.

Muscle flexibility drops by about 5 percent per decade of life, but 10 minutes of stretching every other day can prevent most of this loss as a person ages. Improved flexibility enhances mobility skills, promoting independence by helping older adults perform activities of daily living. Inactive adults continue to gain body fat after age 60, most likely caused by a decrease in basal metabolic rate and physical activity along with increased caloric intake above that required to maintain daily energy requirements.

Older adults who wish to initiate or continue an exercise program are encouraged to have a complete medical exam, including a stress electrocardiogram test. Recommended activities for older adults include calisthenics, walking, jogging, swimming, cycling, and water aerobics. Older adults should avoid isometric and very high-intensity strength-training exercises. Activities that require all-out effort or require participants to hold their breath tend to lessen blood flow to the heart and cause a significant increase in blood pressure and the load placed on the heart. Older adults should participate in activities that require continuous and rhythmic muscular activity (about 40 percent to 60 percent of functional capacity), which do not cause large increases in blood pressure or place an intense overload on the heart.

24) How do I protect myself from quackery and fraud in the fitness/ wellness industry?

The rapid growth in the fitness and wellness industry has unfortunately led to a proliferation of quackery and fraud. Many companies are promoting fraudulent products that make false claims about their ability to provide quick and easy solutions for achieving total well-being. These products include foods, diets, supplements, pills, equipment, books, and videos that are advertised using unproven claims, testimonials, half-truths, and quick-fix statements.

Consumers are often lured by these promises of miraculous results and are willing to pay large sums of money for products that have no scientific basis. Advertisements for these products are not always reliable, as they are often based on unproven claims and testimonials that are meant to appeal to uneducated consumers.

For example, some fitness equipment sold through television and newspaper advertisements may promise to target specific muscle groups and provide quick weight loss results, but these claims are often false. The equipment may be ineffective, and consumers may end up wasting their money on a product that does not work.

Deceit is also found in other sources of information, such as newspaper and magazine articles, trade books, radio, and television shows. Some publishers print books on diets or self-treatment approaches that have no scientific foundation, and reporters may overlook important information or give certain findings greater credence than they deserve.

Consumers must be cautious when seeking health advice on the Internet, as there is a lot of both credible and unconvinced information. It is important to verify the source and credentials of the information. Consumers must be educated and vigilant to avoid falling victim to fraud and quackery in the fitness and wellness industry. It is important to approach health claims with skepticism, do research, and consult with qualified professionals to make informed decisions about your health.

25) What factors should I consider before purchasing exercise equipment?

The author advises readers to carefully consider whether they truly need exercise equipment before making a purchase, as many people buy on impulse and end up with equipment they do not enjoy using and eventually abandon. While some equipment can be valuable for those who prefer indoor exercise, it is important to try out the equipment before purchasing it, and to consider factors such as comfort, stability, and durability. Cheaper brands may not be durable and may be a waste of money. Expensive gadgets such as monitors may be motivating but are not necessary for the actual fitness benefits of the workout and may require costly maintenance. The author suggests seeking advice from professionals and references from people or clubs that have used the equipment extensively. Inexpensive and small equipment such as exercise wheels, skipping ropes, and yoga mats can also provide variety and interest in a workout.

26) What is the greatest benefit of a lifetime wellness lifestyle?

Living an active wellness lifestyle has numerous benefits that can lead to a higher quality of life. By maintaining good health and functional capacity, individuals can avoid sickness and reduce their healthcare expenses and time under medical supervision. Additionally, an active lifestyle can lead to a longer, more productive life. By taking action today and committing to a wellness way of life, we can achieve the freedom to live life to its fullest without limitations. We can also become role models for others and inspire them to adopt a healthier lifestyle. Ultimately, serving mankind is serving God, and by taking care of our bodies and minds, we can contribute to a better world for ourselves and those around us.

You can never step into the same river twice, because new water is always flowing. We are also changing constantly; we are not static sculptures. Jeff Bezos started Amazon in 1994 with a vision to grow like the Amazon River. The arrow in his logo symbolizes that he can deliver anything from A to Z with a smile. if we sincerely believe that we will soon reach the oasis. A boat is safe in the harbour but that is not what the ships are built for. Passion is the only attribute which is infectious. So be passionate about fitness, success is yours.

Happiness is the highest form of health

–**Dalai Lama** (Buddhist Spiritual Leader)

5

Interesting QUOTES

The secret of health for both mind and body are not mourned for the past, not to worry about the future, or not to anticipate troubles, but to line the present moment wisely and earnestly.

–**Siddhartha Gautham Buddha** (Religious leader and Philosopher)

Anything that makes you weak physically intellectually and spiritually reject as poison.

–**Swami Vivekananda** (Hindu Spiritual Leader)

Take up one idea. Make that one idea your life – think of it, dream of it, live on idea. Let the brain, muscles, nerves, every part of your body, be full of that idea, and just leave every other idea alone. This is the way to success.

–**Swami Vivekananda** (Hindu Spiritual Leader)

The attainment of the powerful soul is not possible for a weak individual.

–**Upanishad** (Book-Philosophical Concept of Hinduism)

As wealth is essential for the appropriate fulfillment of desire
Similarly for the salvation of life
Healthy physique is essential.

–**Veda** (Hindu Religious Book)

Be strong, my young friends; that is my advice to you. You will be nearer to Heaven through football than through the study of the Gita. These are bold words; but I have to say them, for I love you. I know where the shoe pinches. You will understand the Gita better with your biceps, your muscles, a little stronger.

–**Swami Vivekanand** (Hindu Spiritual Leader)

Death begins in the colon.

–**Swami Vivekanand** (Hindu Spiritual Leader)

My child I want is muscles of iron and nerves of steel, inside which dwells the mind of the same material as that of which the thunderbolt is made.

–**Swami Vivekananda** (Hindu Spiritual Leader)

A peaceful heart leads to a healthy body; jealousy is like cancer in the bones.

–**Bible** (Proverbs 14:30) (Christian Religious Book)

Do you not know that your body is a temple of the Holy Spirit within you, whom you have from God, and that you are not your own? For you have been purchased at a price. Therefore, glorify God in your body.

–**Bible** (Corinthians 6:19-20) (Christian Religious Book)

A wise man is full of strength, and a man of knowledge enhances his might." "She girds herself with strength; she exerts her arms with vigor.

–Bible (Proverbs 24:5, 31:17) (Christian Religious Book)

Together with a culture of work, there must be a culture of leisure as gratification. To put it another way: people who work must take the time to relax, to be with their families, to enjoy themselves, read, listen to music, play a sport.

–Pope Francis (Former Pope of the Roman Catholic Church)

Ya Allah! Grand me a mind free of worry, a heart free of sadness and a body free of sickness.

–Quran (Islam Religious Book)

There are two blessings which many people waste; Health and Free time.

–Quran (Islam Religious Book)

All mankind is divided into three classes: those that are immovable, those that are movable, and those that move.

–Arab Proverb

Health is digit one, love, glory, happiness and success are zeros. Put the one of health besides the others, you are a rich man. But without the one, everything is zero.

–Arab Proverb

A good laugh and a long sleep are the best cures in the doctor's book.

–Irish proverb

I have two Doctors, my left leg and my right.

–**G.M Trevelyan** (British Historian)

Walking is men's best medicine.

–**Hippocrates** (Greek Philosopher)

A wise man should consider that the health is the greatest of human blessings, and learn by his own thought to derive benefit from his illness.

–**Hippocrates** (Ancient Greek Physician)

As long as your body is healthy and under control, Death is distant, try to save your soul, when death is imminent, what can you do.

–**Chanakya** (Ancient Indian Teacher &Philosopher)

Movement is a medicine for creating change in person's physical, emotional and mental status.

–**Carol Welch** (American Therapeutic Counselor)

A man's health can be judged by which he takes two at a time pills or stairs.

–**Joan Welsh** (American Writer)

An hour of basketball feels like 15 minutes. An hour on a treadmill feels like a weekend in a traffic school.

–**David Walters** (American Politician)

If you think you can or if you think you can't, you are right.

–**Henry Ford** (American Industrialist)

Dance-Great opportunity to kill two birds with one stone-Helps with obesity and health.

–**Nigel Lythgoe** (British Film Director)

If you can't fly, then run
If you can't run, then walk
If you can't walk, then crawl
but whatever you do,
You have to keep moving forward.

–**Martin Luther King Jr.** (American Minister and Nobel Peace Prize Winner)

A part can never be well
Unless the whole is well.

–**Plato** (Athenian Philosopher)

Today, more than 95% of all chronic disease is caused by food choice, toxic food ingredients, nutritional deficiencies and lack of physical exercise.

–**Mike Adams** (American Writer)

Healthy mind in a healthy body.

–**Aristotle** (Greek Philosopher)

We are what we repeatedly do.

–**Aristotle** (Greek Philosopher)

If you want to live a happy life, tie it to a goal. Not to people or things.

–**Albert Einstein** (German Physicist)

Olympism is a philosophy which, by blending sport with culture, seeks to create a way of life based on the joy found in effort, the educational value of good example and respect for universal ethical principles.

–**Juan Antonio Samaranch** (Former International Olympic Committee President)

I believe God created sports for a good reason. It's recreation. It's something that we enjoy. It teaches us a lot as well... I believe God is a sports fan.

–**Paul Rodriguez** (Mexican-American Comedian and Actor)

Sport has the ability to inspire. It has the power to unite people in a way that little else does. It speaks to youth in a language they understand. It is more powerful than Governments. Sport has the power to change the world.

–**Nelson Mandela** (Former President of South Africa)

Doctors are always working to preserve our health and cooks to destroy it, but the later are the more often successful.

–**Denis Diderot** (French philosopher & Writer)

As a father, I believe that involving children in sports at a young age is generally, a wise proposition. I believe that healthy competition is... well. healthy; that sporting events foster a spirit of teamwork that far surpasses the events themselves; and that active participation keeps children moving and is good for their self-esteem.

–**Naveen Jain** (Indian-American Businessman)

Sport is not just about entertainment. It is equally about winning and losing, pooling and galvanizing the energy of the youth, upgrading people's physical fitness and mental prowess.

–**Nita Ambani** (Indian Business Woman & Sports Enthusiast)

Comedy was my sport. It taught me how to roll with the punches. Failure is the exact same as success when it comes to comedy because it just keeps coming. It never stops.

–**Emma Stone** (American Actress)

I am pushing sixty that is enough exercise for me.

–**Mark Twain** (American Author & Humorist)

Gold medals aren't really made of gold. They're made of sweat, determination, and a hard-to-find alloy called guts.

–**Dan Gable** (American Olympic Wrestler &Head Coach)

Fishing is much more than fish. It is the great occasion when we may return to the fine simplicity of our forefathers.

–**Herbert Hoover** (Former President of the United States)

My love for sports will never die. I love martial arts and I want to promote it in whichever way I can. I am a fighter first, then an actor.

–**Akshay Kumar** (Indian Film Actor)

It was easy being healthy when I was young. I was full of energy, so sports and physical challenges were fun. But as I got older and the spring left my step, exercise became harder, and eating, drinking and watching TV became easier. By the time I was 50, I'd put on 50 pounds.

–**Robert Kiyosaki** (American Businessman & Self-Help Author)

I'm a deeply spiritual person, and I strongly believe that God is watching over me!

–**Mahesh Bhupathi** (Indian Tennis Player)

Set a goal, adopt a plan that will help you to achieve the goal. Chances of things happening in this world without goals are slim. Make sure the goal means a lot to you. Believe that the plan is going to win. Tie to people who believe in the plan.

–**Paul "Bear" Bryant** (American Football Player and Coach)

The quality of a person's life is in direct proportion to their commitment to excellence, regardless of their chosen field of endeavour.

–**Vince Lombardi** (American Football Coach)

Courage and confidence are what decision making is all about. It takes courage not only to make decisions, but to live with those decisions afterward.

–**Mike Krzyzewski** (American Basketball Coach)

If you can't afford a doctor, go to an airport-you will get a free x-ray, and a breast exam, and, if you mention Al Qaeda, you'll get a free colonoscopy.

–**Ken baker** (American Journalist)

Health is the greatest of all possessions; a pale cobbler is better than a sick king.

–**Isacc Bickerstaff** (Irish Playwriter)

The food you eat can be the safest form of medicine or the slowest form of poison.

–**Anne wig more** (American Nutritionist)

The Human body is the best work of art.

–Jess C. Scott (American Writer)

Take care of your body. It's the only place you have to live.

–Jim Rohm (American Motivational Speaker)

If a man achieves victory over this body, who in the world can exercise power over him? He who rules himself rules over the whole world.

–Vinoba Bhave (Indian Teacher& Writer).

Health is the thing that makes you feel that now is the best time of the year.

–Franklin Pierce Adams (American Columnist)

Reading is to the mind what exercise is to the body.

–Joseph Addison (English Essayist &Politician.)

Leave all the afternoon for exercise and recreation, which are as necessary as reading. I will rather say more necessary because health is worth more than learning.

–Thomas Jefferson (Former American President)

Jogging is very beneficial. It's good for your legs and your feet. It's also very good for the ground. If makes it feel needed.

–Charles M. Schulz (American Cartoonist)

My wife and I work out together almost every day. It's just a great way to spend time together. We're going to run a marathon together later this year, and that's one more goal that we'll accomplish as husband and wife.

–Bill Rancic (American Entrepreneur)

Our growing softness, our increasing lack of physical fitness, is a menace to our security.

–John F. Kennedy (Former American President)

Early to bed and early to rise makes a man healthy, wealthy and wise.

–Benjamin Franklin (American Scientist & Writer)

To lengthen, thy life; lessen, thy meals.

–Benjamin Franklin (American Scientist & Writer)

It is health that is real wealth and not pieces of gold and silver.

–Mahatma Gandhi (Father of our Nation-India)

We can make a commitment to promote vegetables and fruits and whole grains on every part of every menu. We can make portion sizes smaller and emphasize quality over quantity. And we can help create a culture - imagine this - where our kids ask for healthy options instead of resisting them.

–Michelle Obama (Wife of Former American President Barack Obama & Active Fitness Enthusiast)

I believe that the greatest gift you can give your family and the world is a healthy you.

–Joyce Meyer (American Author & Speaker)

It's so important to realize that every time you get upset, it drains your emotional energy. Losing your cool makes you tired. Getting angry a lot messes with your health.

–Joyce Meyer (American Author & Speaker)

There are shortcuts to happiness and dancing is one of them.

–Vicki Baum (Austrian Writer)

Nothing is so contagious as enthusiasm, it moves stones. It charms brutes.

–**Edward Bulwer –Lytton** (American Football Player & Coach)

You must be true to yourself. Strong enough to be true to yourself. Brave enough to be strong enough to be true to yourself. Wise enough to be brave enough to be strong enough to be shape yourself from what you actually are.

–**Sylvia Constance Ashton-Warner** (New Zealand Poet & Educator)

Do not wait to strike till the iron is hot; but make it hot by striking.

–**William Butler Yeats** (Irish & British Poet)

We don't stop playing because we grow old; we grow old because we stop playing.

–**George Bernard Shaw** (Irish Playwright & Political Activist)

Life must be lived as play.

–**Plato** (Athenian Philosopher)

The greatest mistake in the treatment of diseases is that there are physicians for the body and physicians for the soul, although the two cannot be separated.

–**Plato** (Athenian Philosopher)

Cheerfulness is the best promoter of health and is as friendly to the mind as to the body.

–**Joseph Addison** (English Essayist& Politician)

Healthy citizens are the greatest asset any country can have.

–**Winston S Churchill** (Former Prime Minister UK)

Wine is the most healthful and most hygienic beverages.

–**Louis Pasteur** (French Biologist)

A little chocolate a day keeps the doctor at bay.

–**Marcia Carington** (American Writer)

It is easier to change a man's religion than to change his diet.

–**Margaret Mead** (American Cultural Anthropologist)

The doctor of the future will be oneself.

–**Albert Schweitzer** (French Theologist)

A fit body, a calm mind, a house full of love, these things cannot be bought-they must be earned.

–**Naval Ravikant** (Indian- American Entrepreneur & Investor)

Physical fitness is the first requisite of happiness. In order to achieve happiness, it is imperative to gain mastery of your body. If at the age of 30 you are stiff and out of shape, you are old. If at 60 you are supple and strong then you are young.

–**Joseph Hubertus Pilates** (German Physical Trainer)

Exercise is the closest thing we will ever get to the miracle pill that everyone is seeking. It brings weight loss, appetite control, improved mood, and self-esteem, an energy kick, and longer life by decreasing the risk of heart disease, diabetes, stroke, osteoporosis, and chronic disabilities. Nothing is so contagious as enthusiasm, it moves stones. It charms brutes.

–**Edward Bulwer –Lytton** (Former Parliament Member UK)

Physical fitness is not only one of the most important keys to a healthy body; it is the basis of dynamic and creative intellectual activity.

–**John F. Kennedy** (Former American President)

Life is like riding a bicycle. To keep your balance, you must keep moving.

–**Albert Einstein** (German Physicist)

Sports are the reason I am out of shape. I watch them all on TV.

–**Thomas Sowell** (American Economist)

The dictionary is the only place where success comes before work.

–**Vince Lombardi** (American Football Coach)

Until we decide that we are worth the daily investment in our health, everything else is secondary. We are not destined to pass from the vibrancy and vitality of youth to the frailty of old age unless we choose to.

–**Vonda Wright M.D** (Sports Medicine Specialist)

The more fit you are, the more resilient your brain becomes and the better it functions both cognitively and psychologically. If your body in shape, your mind will follow.

–**John Rately M.D** (American Psychology Professor)

Those who think they have no time for bodily exercise will sooner or later have to find time for illness.

–**Edward Stanley** (British Statesman)

So many people spend their health gaining wealth, and then have to spend their wealth to regain their health.

–A.J Reb Materi (Canadian Clergyman)

Man maintains his balance, poise, and sense of security only as he is moving forward.

–Maxwell Maltz (American Cosmetic Surgeon)

There is difference between interest and commitment. When you are interested in doing something, you do it only when circumstances permit. When you're committed to something, you accept no excuses, only results.

–Art Turock (American Motivational Speaker & Author)

I think it's quite great to set yourself a big challenge, and then you've got another reason for keeping fit.

–Sir Richard Branson (British Businessman & Owner of Virgin Group)

Let him that would move the world, first move himself.

–Socrates (Greek Philosopher)

I don't exercise. If God had wanted me to bend over, he would have put diamonds on the floor.

–Joan Rivers (American Comedian)

I've been on a diet for two weeks and all I've lost is two weeks.

–Totie Fields (American Comedian)

My idea of a balanced diet is a cookie in each hand.

–Barbara Johnson (Judge-Mexico)

I'm not afraid of death. I just don't want to be there when it happens.

–Woody Allen (American film maker)

Movement and rhythm are characteristic of the universe in which we live.

–Lazar Angelov (Bulgarian Fitness Model)

Yoga class helps me calm down from the agonizing stress of trying to get to yoga class on time.

–Sadhguru (Yoga & Educational Expert)

I believe every human has a finite number of heartbeats. I don't intend to waste any of mine running around doing exercises.

–Neil Armstrong (American Astronaut)

Take the admission to the gym to avoid the admission to the hospital.

–Amit Kalantri (Indian Magician & Mentalist)

Many so-called spiritual people, they overeat, drink too much, they smoke and don't exercise. But they do go to church every week and pray, please help my arthritis. Please help me bring up my strength, make me young again.

–Jack LaLanne (American Fitness & Nutrition Expert)

Dying is easy. Living is a pain in the butt. It's like an athletic event. You've got to train for it. You've got to eat right. You've got to exercise. Your health account, your bank account, they're the same thing. The more you put in, the more you can take out.

–Jack LaLanne (American Fitness & Nutrition Expert)

To lose weight, spend time at the gym. To appear like you've lost weight, spend time with people who are bigger than you.

–Mokokoma Mokhonoana (South African Philosopher & Social Critic)

I have to exercise in the morning before my brain figures out what I'm doing.

–Marsha Doble (American Production Director)

Strength does not come from winning. Your struggles develop your strengths. When you go through hardships and decide not to surrender, that is strength.

–Arnold Schwarzenegger (Austrian - American Actor & Body Builder)

The worst thing I can be is the same as everybody else. I hate that.

–Arnold Schwarzenegger (Austrian and American Actor &Body Builder)

The mediocre teacher tells. The good teacher explains

The superior teacher demonstrates: The great teacher inspires.

–William Arthur Ward (American Writer)

We should not judge people by their peak of excellence, but by the distance they have travelled from the point where they started.

–Henry Ward Beecher (American Social Reformer)

smoking is the perfect way to commit suicide without actually dying. According to mark Twain Giving up smoking is easy …I know because I've done it hundreds of times.

–Damien hirst (British Artist)

When performance is measured, performance improves, when performance is measured and reported, the rate of improvement accelerates.

–Thomas S Monson (American Religious Leader & Author)

One cannot think well, love well, sleep well, if one has not dinned well.

–Virgina Wolf (British Writer)

A vigorous five-mile walk will do better for an unhappy but otherwise healthy adult than all the medicine and psychology in the world.

–Paul D white (American Physician)

You are the average of the five people you spend the most time with.

–Jim Rohn (American entrepreneur & motivational speaker)

Everyone thinks of changing the world, but no one thinks of changing himself.

–Tolstoy (Russian Novelist & Anarchist)

Either you run the day or the day runs you.

–Jim Rohn (American Entrepreneur & Motivational Speaker)

The new biology moves us out of victimhood into mastery over our own health.

–**Dr. Bruce Lipton** (American Developmental Biologist)

There is more refreshment and stimulation in a nap, even of the briefest, than in all the alcohol ever distilled.

–**Edward Lucas** (British Writer)

Every man's stomach is like his foot; like one size of shoe does not fit all, one universal diet is not meant for all.

–**Hahne Mann** (German Physician)

Inside me there is a thin person struggling to get out but I usually sedate him with four or five cupcakes.

–**Robert Thaves** (American Cartoonist)

Before thirty, men seek disease; after thirty disease seeks men.

–**Chinese proverb**

To ensure good health: eat lightly breathe deeply, live moderately, cultivate cheerfulness, and maintain an interest in life.

–**William Londen** (British Writer)

Famously joked, my grandmother is over eighty and still doesn't need glasses. Drinks out of the bottle.

–**Henny Youngman** (British-American Comedian & Musician)

We don't stop playing because we grow old; we grow old because we stop playing.

–**George Bernard Shaw** (British Writer)

In order for man to succeed in life, God provided with two means, education and physical activity. Not separately, one for the soul and other for the body, but for the two together. With these means, man can attain perfection

–**Plato** (Greek Philosopher)

Intelligence and skill can only function at the peak of their capacity when the body is healthy and strong.

–**John f Kennedy** (Former American President)

Forty is the old age of youth; fifty is the youth of old age.

–**Victor Hugo** (French Romantic Writer & Politician)

When diet is wrong, medicine is of no use
When diet is correct, medicine is of no need.

–**Ayurvedic proverb**

To eat is divine, but to digest is divine.

–**Ayurvedic proverb**

The age factor means nothing to me. I'm old enough to know my limitations and I'm young enough to exceed them. I'm an 80-year-old rookie. And looking forward to it with boundless enthusiasm.

–**Marv Levy** (American Football Coach)

Age is a case of mind over matter. If you don't mind, it doesn't matter. How old would you be if you didn't know how old you are?

–**Leroy Satchel Paige** (American Baseball Player)

Work like you don't need the money. Love like you've never been hurt. Dance like nobody's watching.

–**Leroy Satchel Paige** (American Baseball Player)

Be strong in body, clean in mind, lofty in ideals.

–**James Naismith** (Canadian American Physical Educator-Inventor of Basketball)

You can't live a perfect day without doing something for someone who will never be able to repay you.

–**John Wooden** (American Basketball Coach)

Some people want it to happen, some wish it would happen, others make it happen.

–**Michael Jordan** (American Basketball Player)

Always remember, anything is yours if you are willing to pay the price.... One hundred percent is not enough.

–**George Allen** (American Football Coach)

The quality of a person's life is in direct proportion to their commitment to excellence, regardless of their chosen field of endeavor.

–**Vince Lombardi** (American Football Coach)

The answer is surprisingly simple. Just do right. Live an honorable life. Do your best. Treat others as you want to be treated.

–**Lou Holtz** (American Football Player &Coach)

Confidence builds slowly, but once you get there, confidence breeds confidence.

–**Marv Levy** (American Football Coach)

To be successful, you don't have to do extraordinary things. Just do ordinary things extraordinarily well.

–**John Rohn** (American Basketball Player)

He doesn't know the meaning of the word fear, but then again, he doesn't know the meaning of most words.

–**Bobby Bowden** (American Football Coach)

Success is never final. Failure is never fatal. It's courage that counts.

–**John Wooden** (American Basketball Player &Coach)

If you shoot for the stars and hit the moon, it's OK. But you've got to shoot for something. A lot of people don't even shoot.

–**Robert Townsend** (American Comedian &Writer)

We should never discourage young people from dreaming dreams.

–**Lenny Wilkens** (American Basketball Player)

You find that you have peace of mind and can enjoy yourself, get more sleep, rest when you know that it was a 100 percent effort that you gave—win or lose.

–**Gordie Howe** (Canadian Ice Hockey Player)

Leaders are made, they are not born. They are made by hard effort, which is the price which all of us must pay to achieve any goal that is worthwhile.

–**Vince Lombardi** (American Football Player &Coach)

There are not traffic jams along the extra mile.

–**Roger Staubach** (American Football Player)

I'm an early guy and a late guy.

–**Ray Rhodes** (American Football Player)

Winning is only half of it. Having fun winning is the other half.

–**Bum Phillips** (American Football Coach)

If you're bored with life—you don't get up every morning with a burning desire to do things—you don't have enough goals.

–**Lou Holtz** (American Football Player)

Don't let other people tell you what you want.

–**Pat Riley** (American Basketball Player & Executive)

Self-praise is for losers. Be a winner. Stand for something. Always have class, and be humble.

–**John Madden** (American Football Coach)

A successful leader has to be innovative. If you are not one step ahead of the crowd, you'll soon be a step behind everyone else.

–**Tom Landry** (American Football Player & Coach)

Don't go to the grave with life unused.

–**Bobby Bowden** (American Football Coach)

Life is 10 percent what happens to you and 90 percent how you respond to it.

–**Lou Holtz** (American Football Player)

The harder you work, the luckier you get.

–**Gary Player** (South African Golfer)

Management must speak with one voice. When it doesn't, management itself becomes a peripheral opponent to the team's mission.

–**Pat Riley** (American Basketball Coach &Executive)

Praise is a great motivator. Criticism is a great teaching tool if done properly, but praise is the best motivator.

–**John Wooden** (American Basketball Coach)

You're never a loser until you quit trying.

–**Mike Ditka** (American Football Player)

A winner never stops trying.

–**Tom Landry** (American Football Player)

Winners never quit and quitters never win.

–**Vince Lombardi** (American Football Coach)

Difficulties in life are intended to make us better, not bitter.

–**Dan Reeves**, (American Football Coach)

It may sound strange, but many champions are made champions by setbacks.

–**Bob Richards** (American Athlete & Minister)

There's no great fun, satisfaction, or joy from doing something that's easy.

–**John Wooden**, (American Basketball Coach)

Paralyze resistance with persistence.

–**Woody Hayes** (American Football Coach)

It's just a job. Grass grows, birds fly, waves pound the sand. I beat people up.

–**Muhammad Ali** (American Boxer)

You're never as good as everyone tells you when you win, and you're never as bad as they say when you lose.

–**Lou Holtz** (American Football Coach)

Winning is overrated. The only time it is really important is in surgery and war.

–**Al McGuire** (American Basketball Coach)

When you are younger you get blamed for crimes you never committed and when you're older you begin to get credit for virtues you never possessed.

–**Casey Stengel** (American Baseball Player)

The power of the human will to compete and the drive to excel beyond the body's normal capabilities is most beautifully demonstrated in the arena of sport.

–**Aimee Mullins** (American Para Olympian Athlete & Actress)

To give yourself the best possible chance of playing to your potential, you must prepare for every eventuality. That means practice.

–**Seve Ballesteros** (Spanish Golfer)

Good, better, best. Never let it rest. Until your good is better and your better is best.

–**Tim Duncan** (American Basketball Player)

The key is not the will to win... everybody has that. It is the will to prepare to win that is important. Everyone wants to be on a winning team, but no one wants to come to practice.

–**Bobby Knight** (American Basketball Player)

It's not necessarily the amount of time you spend at practice that counts; it's what you put into practice that makes the difference.

–**Eric Lindros**, (American Hockey Coach)

The difference between a good athlete and a top athlete is the top athlete will do the mundane things when nobody's looking.

–**Susan True** (American Leader)

If you train hard, you'll not only be hard, you'll be hard to beat.

–**Herschel Walker** (American Football Player)

Publicity is like poison. It doesn't hurt unless you swallow it.

–**Joe Paterno** (American Football Player & Manager)

All quitters are good losers.

–**Bob Zuppke** (American Football Coach)

Be more concerned with your character than your reputation, because your character is what you really are, while your reputation is merely what others think you are.

–**John Wooden** (American Basketball Coach)

Every one of our players respects every one of their players and their team as a whole. But once we cross that white line most of the respect will be out the window and we will be fighting to win the game.

–**David Beckham** (English Soccer Player)

If anything goes bad, I did it. If anything goes semi-good, then we did it. If anything goes really well, then you did it. That's all it takes to get people to win football games.

–**Paul "Bear" Bryant** (American Football Player)

Everybody wants to take responsibility when you win, but when you fail, all these fingers are pointing.

–**Mike Krzyzewski** (American Basketball Coach)

A manager doesn't hear the cheers.

–**Alvin Dark** (American Baseball Coach)

Either love your players or get out of coaching.

–**Bobby Dodd** (American Football Player & Coach)

Praise your kids. Inspire and motivate your players with praise. Ten years from now it won't matter what your record was. Will your kids love you or hate you?

–**Jim Harrick** (American Basketball Coach)

I believe managing is like holding a dove in your hand. If you hold it too tightly you kill it, but if you hold it too loosely, you lose it.

–**Tommy Lasorda** (American Baseball Player & Coach)

You can motivate by fear, and you can motivate by reward. But both those methods are only temporary. The only lasting thing is self-motivation.

–**Homer Rice** (American Football Player & Coach)

I never criticize a player unless they are convinced of my unconditional confidence in them.

–**John Robinson** (American Football Player & Coach)

The principle is competing against yourself. It's about self-improvement, about being better than you were the day before.

–Steve Young (American Football Player)

I think the biggest asset of successful people is that they are not afraid of success. There are so many people who are afraid of having success for fear of having to repeat their successful ways. It's so easy to see that in people. I'll read quotes in the newspaper, and I can tell people who are afraid to be good.

–Mike Bossy (Canadian Ice Hockey Player)

Success is not the result of spontaneous combustion. You must first set yourself on fire.

–Fred Shero (Canadian Ice Hockey Player)

The strong take from the weak and the smart take from the strong.

–Pete Carril (American Basketball Coach)

Nothing devastates a football team like a selfish player. It's a cancer.

–Paul Brown (American Football Coach)

It's amazing how much can be accomplished if no one cares about who gets the credit.

–Blanton Collier (American Football Coach)

Good teams become great ones when the members trust each other enough to surrender the Me for the We.

–Phil Jackson (American Basketball Player)

Teamwork is the ability to have different thoughts about things. It's the ability to argue and stand up and say loud and strong what you feel. But in the end, it's also the ability to adjust to what is the best for the team.

–**Tom Landry** (American Football Player)

There's nothing greater in the world than when somebody on the team does something good, and everybody gathers around to pat him on the back.

–**Billy Martin** (American Baseball Player)

The secret is to work less as individuals and more as a team. As a coach, I play not my eleven best, but my best eleven. Most football players are temperamental. That's 90 percent temper and 10 percent mental.

–**Doug Plank** (American Football Player & Coach)

There is an old saying about the strength of the wolf is the pack, and I think there is a lot of truth to that. On a football team, it's not the strength of the individual players, but it is the strength of the unit and how they all function together.

–**Bill Belichick** (American Football Coach)

If you get the best players, you're going to get the kids who have egos. You have to take the 'I' concept out and get the 'we' concept.

–**Bobby Bowden** (American Football Coach)

Don't tell your problems to people: 80 percent don't care, and the other 20 percent are glad you have them.

–**Lou Holtz** (American Football Coach)

It is better to be devoured by lions than to be eaten by dogs.

–**Alex Agase** (American Football Player)

I don't want a team that escapes from reality and escapes from the truth. I don't want people who are always escaping, who always have a story and are always conniving. An ostrich tries to escape from the truth. Isn't an ostrich the thing that puts its head in the sand? But guess what's sticking out when he does it? It's ass, that's what. I don't want a team like that. Because when you have a team like that and trouble comes, that team will not face the trouble.

–**John Chaney** (American Basketball Coach)

The values learned on the playing field-how to set goals, endure, take criticism and risks, become team players, use our bodies, stay healthy and deal with stress-prepare us for life.

–**Donna de Varona** (American Swimmer)

Always turn a negative situation into a positive situation. My attitude is that if you push me towards something that you think is a weakness, then I will turn that perceived weakness into a strength.

–**Michael Jordan** (American Basketball Player)

The difference between a successful person and others is not lack of strength, not a lack of knowledge, but rather a lack of will.

–**Vince Lombardi** (American Football Coach)

A winner has dedication and pride and the will to win, and he'll do a little bit extra every day to improve himself and his winning team. A winner is worried about his team and his school, and he'll outwork people, and he'll sacrifice.

–**Paul "Bear" Bryant** (American Football Player & Coach)

First become a winner in life. Then it's easier to become a winner on the field.

–Tom Landry (American Football Player &Coach)

Everything looks nicer when you win. The girls are prettier. The cigars taste better. The trees are greener.

–Billy Martin (American Baseball Player)

Happiness is a good bank account, a good cook, and a good digestion.

–Jean-Jacques Rousseau (Genevan Philosopher)

I always say, 'Eat clean to stay fit; have a burger to stay sane.'

–Gigi Hadid (American Model)

The most important thing is to try and inspire people so that they can be great in whatever they want to do.

–Kobe Bryant (American Basketball Player)

Math is like going to the gym for your brain. It sharpens your mind.

–Danica McKellar (American Actress)

Exercise is really important to me - it's therapeutic. So, if I'm ever feeling tense or stressed or like I'm about to have a meltdown, I'll put on my iPod and head to the gym or out on a bike ride along Lake Michigan with the girls.

–Michelle Obama (Former First Lady of United States)

The first duties of the physician is to educate the masses not to take medicine.

–William Osler (Canadian Physician)

Exercise should be regarded as the tribute to the heart

–**Gene Tunney** (American Boxer)

God heals and doctor takes the fee

–**Benjamin Franklin** (Founding Father of the United States)

You cannot teach a person anything
You can only help him to find it for himself

–**Galileo** (Italian Physicist)

Smile And Let Everyone Know That Today, you're a Lot Stronger Than You Were Yesterday

–**Jelly** (Dutch Youtuber)

Your body is what makes your sexy. Your smile is what make you pretty. But your personality makes you beautiful.

–**Adriana Lima** (Brazilian Model)

Your Body Hears Everything Your Mind Has to Say

–**Sarah Fragoso** (Australian journalist)

A healthy attitude is contagious, but don't wait to catch it from others. Be a carrier

–**Tom Stoppard** (Czech-born British Playwright and Screenwriter)

Happiness is not determined by what's happening around you, but rather what's happening inside you

–**John Spence** (American Musician)

The physical body is not only a temple for our soul, but the means by which we embark on the inward journey toward the core.

–**B.K.S. Iyengar** (Indian Yoga Guru and Author)

My Body Is My Temple and Asanas Are My Prayers

–**B.K.S. Iyengar** (Indian Yoga Guru and Author)

Action is movement with intelligence. The world is filled with movement. What the world needs is more conscious movement, more action.

–**B.K.S. Iyengar** (Indian Yoga Guru and Author)

Yoga is a light, which once lit, will never dim. The better your practice, the brighter the flame.

–**B.K.S. Iyengar** (Indian Yoga Guru and Author)

The attainment of a powerful soul is not possible for a weak individual

–**Upanishad** (Hindu Religious Book)

You cannot buy it, you can't read it, you have to earn it. My formula has always been: love yourself, move your body, watch your portions

–**Jean Nidetch** (American Fitness Expert)

Earth has the resources to meet everyone's needs, but not everyone's greed.

–**Mahatma Gandhi** (Father of the Nation -India)

Our stomachs should not be a graveyard for other animals

–**Philip Wollen** (Australian philanthropist)

A playground may not be considered like a church, but it is also not like a bar

–**Frank Lautenberg** (US senator)

Winners are like kites, they rise highest against the wind, not with it

–**Winston Churchill** (Former Prime Minister of UK)

The food you eat can be either the safest and most powerful form of medicine or the slowest form of poison

–**Ann Wigmore** (US Health Practitioner)

Only one who devotes himself to a cause with his whole strength and soul can be a true master. For this reason, mastery demands all of a person

–**Albert Einstein** (German-born theoretical physicist)

The greatest discovery of my generation is that a human being can alter his life by altering his attitudes

–**William James** (American philosopher and psychologist)

A merry heart doeth good like a medicine, but a broken spirit drieth the bones in the Bible

–**Bible** (Book of Proverbs 17:22)

What fits your busy schedule better, exercising one hour a day or being dead 24 hours a day

–**Randy Pausch** (Professor of Computer Science, USA)

Never, under any circumstances, take a sleeping pill and a laxative on the same night

–**Dave Barry** (American comedian)

The only reason I exercise is so that I can eat more

–**Mark Twain** (American comedian and actor)

Thought-Provoking Quotes with Unknown Authors

- Cut carbs? Sure, I can do that.... slices bread.
- My body is a temple where junk food goes to worship.
- My favourite exercise is a cross between a lunge and a crunch, I call it Lunch.
- Sweat is your fat crying.
- I am on a seafood diet; I see food and I eat it.
- Girl you are my cardio. You get my heart racing.
- The only exercise some people get is jumping to conclusions, running down their friends, side-stepping responsibility and pushing their luck.
- Rabbit hops all day, only eat vegetables, but only live 5 years. Whales swim all day, only drink water, but are fat Tortoise do nothing energetic but live for 250 years. And you tell me to exercise? I do not think so.
- I tried exercise but found I was allergic to it. My skin flushed, my heart raced, I got sweaty and short of breath. Very dangerous.
- I'm not overweight. I'm just under tall.
- I have a condition that prevents me from going on a diet... I get hungry.
- I have a love-hate relationship with my body. Currently, we're on a break.
- I tried to do yoga, but I kept falling asleep in corpse pose.

- My idea of a perfect workout is one that involves lying down and not moving for an extended period of time.
- I don't have a problem with caffeine. I have a problem without it.
- I don't always go to the gym, but when I do, I make sure everyone knows about it on social media.
- My doctor told me to start exercising. I told him I already do. He asked me what I do. I said, 'Well, I lift weights... occasionally I lift my feet to put on my shoes
- I'm not out of shape, I'm just experiencing a bulking phase.
- I don't need a personal trainer. My anxiety provides me with enough cardio.
- I'm not lazy, I'm just on energy-saving mode.
- I don't jog. It makes the ice jump out of my glass.
- I hate it when I go to the gym and forget my motivation at home.
- I don't have a six-pack, but I do have a keg.
- I tried to catch some fog earlier, but I mist.
- Don't forget to exercise your funny bone. Laughter is the best medicine, so make sure to watch some funny videos or tell some jokes every day.
- If you're feeling stressed, take a deep breath and remind yourself that nothing is more important than your health. Except maybe pizza.
- The only running I do is running late.

- Don't forget to stretch before and after your workout, or you'll be walking like a robot for the next few days.
- When I exercise, I wear all black it's a funeral for my fat
- "I" is the only difference between fit and fat
- I thought they said "rum"
- I consider my refusal to go to Gym today as resistance training
- My favourite machine at the gym is the television.
- Education is important, but big biceps are importanter.
- Excuses don't burn calories. Push ups do!
- The best abs exercise is five sets of stops eating so much.
- He refers to the human bloodstream as a "River of Life," which is "polluted" by "junk foods" loaded with preservatives, salt, sugar, and artificial flavourings.
- Crying-is an emotional safety valve that opens when the inner pressure is too great to handle.
- Exercise is the poor man's plastic surgery
- Sports for all: All for sports
- Sitting is injurious to health, sitting is new smoking
- A belly full of laughs is a hot belly indeed
- Disease-dis-ease-Lack of ease or balance
- Our gut is the second brain of the body
- Diet is not a sprint, it's a marathon

- S4D-Sports for Development
- The flatter the TV the rounder your stomach.
- Fitness can neither be bought nor bestowed. Like honor, it must be earned
- When 'I' is replaced by 'We'-Even Illness Becomes "Wellness"
- If you live a healthy life style from birth you might live hundred years or beyond, start from twenty years of age, A century might still be around. Alas! for every year after this you will lose a year and a half. And starting beyond the fifties you start with a handicap. So, pray God.
- The body heals with play, the mind heals with laughter and the spirit heals with joy.
- Give a man a soccer ball, he plays for a moment. Teach a man to play soccer, he plays for the life time.
- Exercise equals endorphins. Endorphins make you happy
- Physical activity is something you do, physical fitness is something you acquire, a characteristic or an attribute one can achieve by being physically active. And exercise is structured and tends to have fitness as its goal
- I am trying to fit 30 minutes of daily exercise into my busy schedule. Today I took 120 fifteen –second Walks.
- Get fit, in the gym; lose weight in the kitchen.
- Have fun, when you work out; And it won't feel, Like work.
- Every time you, Eat or drink; You are either, feeding disease or fighting it.

- A weak person who has a weak body or a weak mind can never be master of a strong soul.
- Do not pray for an easy life, pray for the strength.
- Seeking happiness for others, you find it for yourself.
- Laugh it up | Just move it
- Stress less day |Fitness Bee
- The gym, where fat is burned; and pride is earned.
- If it doesn't challenge you; it doesn't change you
- Laziness fuels, more laziness; activity fuels, more activity
- Families that exercise together, stay together.
- I have a love-hate relationship with my gym. We break up every couple of months, but then we get back together.
- I always start my diet on the same day every year - tomorrow.
- The older you get, the tougher it is to lose weight because by then, your body and your fat have become really good friends.
- Laughter is the best medicine. Unless you have diarrhoea.
- Only a master Gardner knows how much water, fertilizer and pruning a plant needs. In the same way, if we are not masters, we should not prune our children, lest we cut off some essential part that may never grow back.
- The only time I ever run is when I'm late for pizza.
- Going to the gym is like paying rent for your muscles, except your landlord is a personal trainer, who's always asking for more.

- For good health, be mindful of both the things going through your mouth and the things coming out from your mouth
- Pressure, Sugar, Cholesterol (PSC) - The three letters you don't want to hear from your doctor, unless it stands for Pizza, Sushi, and Chocolate - then it's just a delicious meal plan.
- The finger raise of the umpire in cricket is not interesting for the batsman, but it is very much interesting for the bowler
- Creative coaches are like willow trees, bending under forceful winds, while stiff coaches are like pine trees - they break under strong winds.
- Children are like sunflowers, naturally inclined to lean towards the warmth and nourishment of love, affection, and protection.
- I wish I could turn my fat into muscle, but apparently, it's not that easy. It's like turning lead into gold, but with more sweat.
- Eating healthy is important, but don't forget to indulge in your favourite treats once in a while. Life is short, so enjoy the occasional slice of pizza or chocolate cake.
- Don't forget to stretch your legs, especially when binge-watching your favourite TV show. Get up and do some jumping jacks during commercial breaks.
- Practice good hygiene, but don't become a germaphobe. It's okay to touch a doorknob or shake hands with someone.
- Remember to get enough sleep, but don't oversleep. The early bird may get the worm, but the late owl gets the extra snooze time.

- Finally, always remember that an apple a day keeps the doctor away. But a glass of wine a day keeps the stress away. Cheers to good health!

- If you're feeling too lazy to work out, just remember that "sweatpants" is a formal term for athletic wear.

- Laugh often. Laughter is the best medicine, and it's also a great ab workout!

- Dance like nobody's watching. It doesn't matter if you have two left feet or if you're a professional dancer, just put on some music and move your body!

- Drink plenty of water, but also treat yourself to a nice glass of wine or a delicious cocktail every now and then. Life is all about balance, right?

- Take naps. Naps are not just for kids, they're for adults too! Plus, you'll be less grumpy after a good nap.

- Hug a friend (or a pet). Hugs release oxytocin, the "feel-good" hormone, and they're a great way to show someone you care.

- Eat your veggies, but also indulge in some pizza, ice cream, or other guilty pleasures once in a while. Just remember, moderation is key.

- Exercise regularly, but don't forget to rest and recover. Your body needs time to recharge, just like your phone.

- Spend time outdoors. Fresh air and sunshine can do wonders for your mood and your health. Plus, you might even spot some cute animals!

- Don't take life too seriously. Sometimes you just need to laugh at yourself and embrace your silly side.

- Practice gratitude. Even on your worst days, there's always something to be thankful for. Plus, it's a great excuse to treat yourself to some chocolate.
- Sitting can be injurious to health
- Consistency is more important than intensity
- Enjoyment is the key factor, when we get older
- The body heals with play, the mind heals with laughter and sprit heals with joy
- Laughing is internal jogging
- If you have time for social media, then you have time for exercise
- We rest we rust
- Exercise thy lasting youth defends
- Exercise is not the fountain of youth: it is good drink of vitality
- Just as pooled water tends to accumulate impurities, the human blood also requires proper circulation through exercise to stay healthy.
- No need to run marathon, take stairs, gardening, walking with dogs for fitness
- Resistance training is the best
- Exercise produces myokines that improves intellectual function
- Sit on the floor more often for flexible lower body
- Train insane or remain the same
- One meal won't make you healthy just like one workout won't make you healthy

- Don't limit your challenges; challenge your limits
- Train like a beast; look like a beauty
- Be stronger than your excuses
- The more you train; the bigger your smile
- At first, they'll ask why you're doing it. later, they'll ask how you did it
- Don't tell people your plans, show them your results
- Wish less work more
- Exercise and gym are the greatest anti-depressants in the world
- I got 99 problems, but I'm going to the gym to ignore all of them.
- Quitting is never an option unless you want to make it a habit.
- Your body can handle almost anything, you simply need to convince your mind.
- Focusing on your health and wellness is the best investment you can ever make.
- Next year around the same time, you will thank yourself for starting your fitness journey.
- Brave, bold men, these are what we want. What we want is vigour in the blood, strength in the nerves, iron muscles and nerves of steel, not softening namby-pamby ideas. Avoid all these. Avoid all mystery.
- The highest manifestation of strength is to keep ourselves calm and on our own feet.

- The remedy for weakness is not brooding over weakness, but thinking of strength.
- Fitness is a journey, not a race, or a sprint
- What's impossible today, will be your warm-up tomorrow.
- The spinal cord that links between the brain and the body
- Exercise is a double-edged weapon. fit people are large hearted because the heart size has increased (hypertrophy).
- If you are don't stretch your muscles, you are stretching your luck.
- The internal rhythms, the inherent clockwork-like nature of the nervous and endocrine systems, have become unbalanced through the effects of stress and tension, resulting in feeling of discomfort and lack of wellbeing. And leading to disease and neurosis
- The only difference with white people and black is in the percentage of melanin
- Employees build organizations, fitter the employees, the better will be the organization. If you love your job-you don't have to work for a single day in your life
- Our foot has many nerve endings, which get smoothened when contact with natural grass and sand.
- Wake up stretches will activate your spine and body -watch the cat or dog waking up from sleep, they do one or two stretches before start to run
- Every drug that has an effect has a side effect but physical activity has only positive effect. Walking 2 kilometres in 20

minutes for adult, slow... fast... slow... read paper or TV after walk for relaxation

- London has it where you pay extra for driving during peak hours and invest the revenue generated in public transport. Singapore taxes cars in a big way to deter car ownership. Such polices are good for energy saving, causes less traffic and more physical activity
- Humans were born with a tail remember? We lost our tail because we never used it. we might soon lose out on our muscles and bone density, as we just don't seem to use either of these live tissues
- Strength training will not reduce weight- Muscle weigh 5-7 times more than fat-during the weight training fat will convert to muscle mass. The increased muscle mass can cause better metabolism. The aim of our fitness training must be reducing the unwanted fat and increasing muscle mass.
- Human body is a wonderful creation of God. He has installed the software to reboot whenever in need. You have to be literate enough to operate this machine.
- Be more than yesterday and less than tomorrow
- Sleep is that golden chain that ties health and our bodies together
- Better sore than sorry
- Biceps don't grow on trees
- Eat less CRAP

  C-Carbonated Drinks

  R-Refined Sugar

A-Artificial sweeteners and colours

P-Processed foods

- Eat more FOOD

F-Fruits and Vegetables

O-Organic lean protein

O-Omega 3 fatty acids

D-Drink Water

Few Jokes

1. A minister was the chief guest at the finals of a football tournament. After giving away the prizes, he was requested to say a few words. He said, it pains me to learn that this year only two teams could make it to the finals. When we have hundreds of football clubs in the country, we should endeavour to see that many more teams reach the finals next year.

2. A Fitness Enthusiast went to the doctor to get some medicine as he was not feeling well. This is pretty strong stuff, said the doctor, so take some the first day, then skip a day, take some again on the third day and skip another day and so on. A few months later the doctor met the Sardarji's wife and asked how he was.

   Oh, he is dead, she told him.

   Did not the medicine I prescribed do him any good? Asked the doctor

   Oh, the medicine was all right, she replied. It was all the skipping that killed him.

3. During the selections for the school football team, the coach gave the players the option for selecting their own playing positions. The players made up their minds and the coach began to ask them about their playing positions: The conversation went as follows:

   Coach: Banerjee?

   Banerjee: Centre Forward, Sir.

   Coach: Kumar?

   Kumar: Right back sir

   Coach: What about you Singh?

   Singh: There is a slight problem

   Coach: What?

   Singh: My friends are wicked; they want me to play Left Out Sir.

   Coach: So, what's the problem?

   Singh: How can I play left out? Won't I have to play outside the field, sir?

4. Once upon a time, there was an athlete who had set her sights on winning the gold medal in the world championship for long jump. Sadly, she didn't quite make it and missed out on the top spot. The next day, a newspaper headline screamed, "Athlete Loses Gold Medal in Long Jump!" Now, our dear sports minister, who was very inferior in knowledge, read this news and got really puzzled. He stated, she must have taken the jump after removing the gold.

6

Fitness tips

Methods to improve physical fitness and nutrition

- Use social media to share information and tips about physical fitness and nutrition.
- Host community events, such as a walk-a-thon or healthy cooking classes, to promote healthy behaviors.
- Partner with local schools to teach students about the importance of physical activity and proper nutrition.
- Host webinars or virtual workshops to share information about healthy lifestyle habits.
- Create an online forum or support group for individuals interested in improving their physical fitness and nutrition.
- Use billboards or other outdoor advertising to promote healthy habits.

- Offer free or discounted gym memberships or nutrition counselling to encourage individuals to try new healthy behaviours.
- Partner with local restaurants to offer healthy menu options or host healthy cooking competitions.
- Host charity events, such as a fun run, to raise awareness and funds for physical fitness and nutrition education.
- Host a healthy food drive to collect and donate nutritious food to local food banks or shelters.
- Work with healthcare providers to offer health screenings and educational resources to patients.
- Offer employee wellness programs in the workplace, such as lunchtime yoga classes or healthy cooking workshops.
- Partner with local sports teams to promote physical activity and healthy lifestyles.
- Organize a community garden or other outdoor activity space for individuals to use for physical activity.
- Offer virtual or in-person personal training sessions or group fitness classes.
- Provide incentives or rewards for individuals who engage in healthy behaviors, such as discounts on gym memberships or healthy meal delivery services.
- Host a health fair to provide education and resources on physical fitness and nutrition.
- Use storytelling or personal testimonies to inspire and motivate individuals to make healthy lifestyle changes.
- Work with local media outlets to share information about physical fitness and nutrition.

- Collaborate with community leaders and organizations to create a culture of health and wellness in the community.

Technology for physical fitness

- Wearable technology: Wearable technology such as fitness trackers, smartwatches, and heart rate monitors can be used to track physical activity and monitor progress towards fitness goals.
- Virtual reality: Virtual reality can be used to create immersive fitness experiences, such as virtual exercise classes, to make workouts more engaging and fun.
- Mobile apps: Mobile apps can provide personalized workout plans and track progress, making it easier for individuals to stay on track with their fitness goals.
- Artificial intelligence: Artificial intelligence can be used to create personalized workout plans based on an individual's fitness level, goals, and preferences.
- Smart gym equipment: Smart gym equipment can track performance and provide real-time feedback to individuals, helping them to optimize their workouts.
- Gamification: Gamification can be used to make physical fitness more fun and engaging, such as turning workouts into games that incentivize individuals to push themselves harder.
- Augmented reality: Augmented reality can be used to enhance workout experiences, such as providing real-time coaching and feedback during exercises.
- Biometric sensors: Biometric sensors can track vital signs such as heart rate and breathing rate, providing valuable information to individuals and trainers.

- Social media: social media can be used to connect with like-minded individuals and build a community around physical fitness, providing support and motivation.

- Online coaching: Online coaching can provide personalized fitness plans and coaching to individuals, no matter where they are in the world.

- 3D printing: 3D printing can be used to create customized equipment and prosthetics that are tailored to an individual's body and fitness needs.

- Robotics: Robotics can be used to create advanced exercise equipment that adapts to an individual's movements and provides resistance tailored to their strength level.

- Machine learning: Machine learning can be used to analyze and optimize workout data, providing individuals with insights on how to improve their performance.

- Biofeedback: Biofeedback can be used to provide real-time feedback on an individual's physical state, helping them to better understand their body and optimize their workouts.

- Virtual coaches: Virtual coaches can provide personalized feedback and coaching to individuals during workouts, helping them to stay motivated and on track.

- Wearable resistance training: Wearable resistance training can provide resistance during workouts without the need for bulky equipment, making it easier to exercise anywhere.

- Haptic technology: Haptic technology can provide tactile feedback during workouts, helping individuals to better understand their body's movements and optimize their form.

- Brain-computer interfaces: Brain-computer interfaces can be used to control exercise equipment using the power of the mind, creating a more immersive and engaging workout experience.
- Exergaming: Exergaming combines video games with physical activity, making workouts more fun and engaging for individuals of all ages.

Improving nutritional value of food without enhancing the home budget

- Cook at home instead of eating out. This allows you to control the quality of the ingredients and the amount of salt, sugar, and fat in your meals.
- Buy in bulk. You can save money by purchasing larger quantities of staple foods like rice, beans, and oats.
- Use cheaper cuts of meat. Lean meats like chicken breast and sirloin steak are expensive. Try using less expensive cuts of meat like ground beef or pork shoulder.
- Make your own meals instead of buying pre-packaged foods. Homemade meals are generally healthier and less expensive than pre-packaged foods.
- Buy seasonal produce. Fruits and vegetables that are in season are often less expensive than those that are out of season.
- Use frozen fruits and vegetables. They are usually cheaper than fresh produce and can be just as nutritious.

- Choose whole grains over refined grains. Whole grains are more filling and provide more nutrients than refined grains like white bread and pasta.
- Use plant-based protein sources. Legumes like beans and lentils are a great source of protein and are often less expensive than meat.
- Shop at discount stores or ethnic markets. They often offer lower prices on produce, meats, and grains.
- Use herbs and spices instead of salt to add flavour to your meals. This can help reduce your salt intake and save you money.
- Plan your meals ahead of time. This helps you avoid impulsive purchases and reduces food waste.
- Use leftovers. Leftovers can be turned into new meals and can save you money on groceries.
- Drink water instead of sugary drinks. Water is healthier and cheaper than soda and juice.
- Avoid processed and packaged foods. These are often high in salt, sugar, and fat and can be expensive.
- Use smaller plates. This can help you control portion sizes and reduce food waste.
- Grow your own herbs and vegetables. This can be a fun and rewarding way to save money on produce.
- Buy generic brands. Generic brands are often less expensive than name-brand products and can be just as good.
- Eat slowly and mindfully. This can help you enjoy your meals more and reduce overeating.

7

Images

1. More Playgrounds are Needed than Hospitals

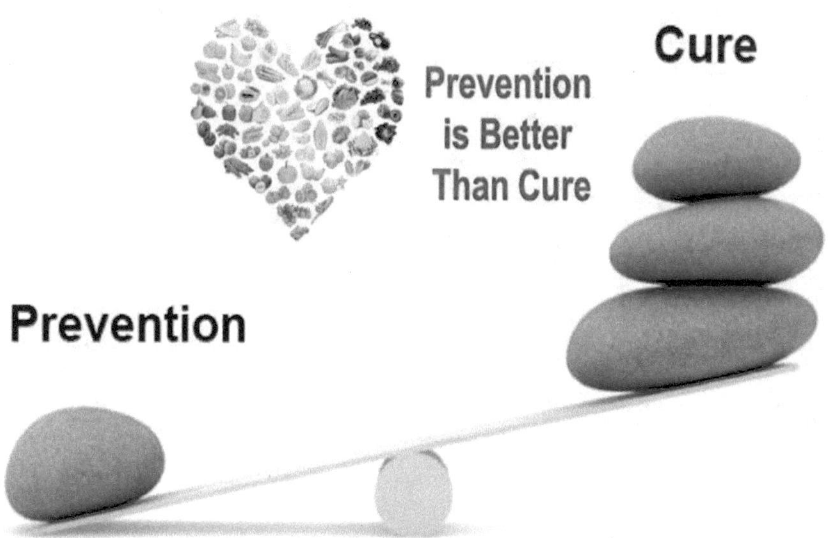

2. Becoming Wider is Easy

Why am I getting older
and wider instead of
older and wiser???

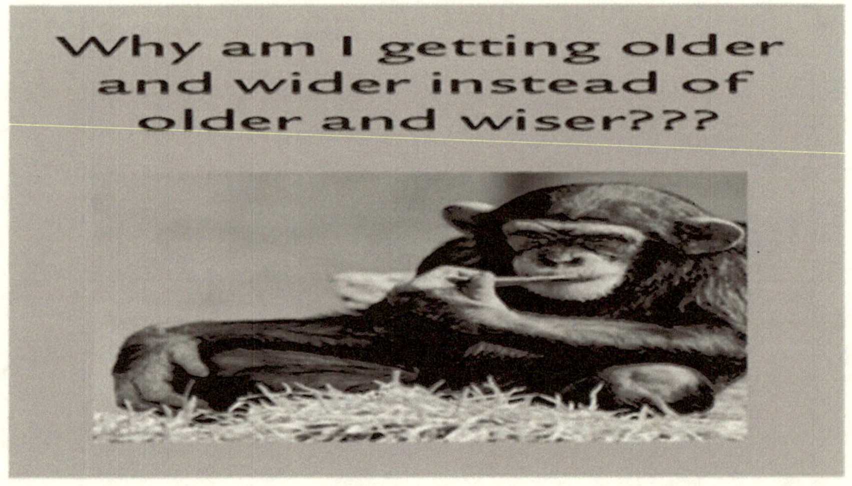

3. Combination of Exercise and Diet for Fitness

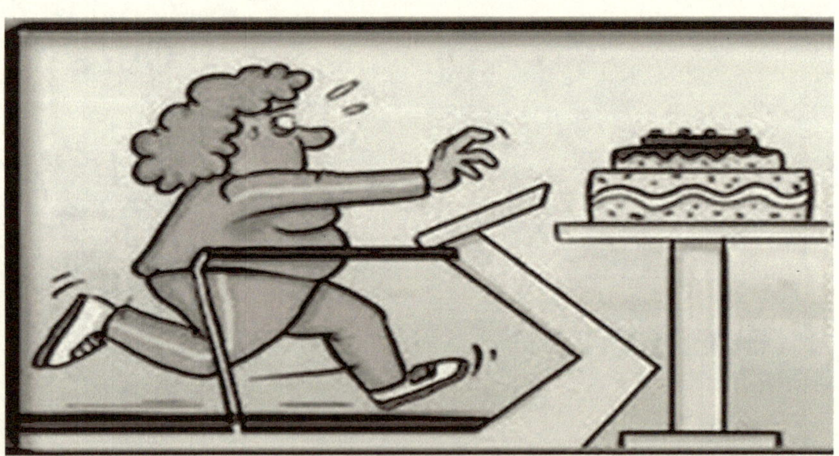

4. Consistent Dream of Fitness for Attainment of Goal

CONSISTENCY IS MORE
IMPORTANT THAN INTENSITY

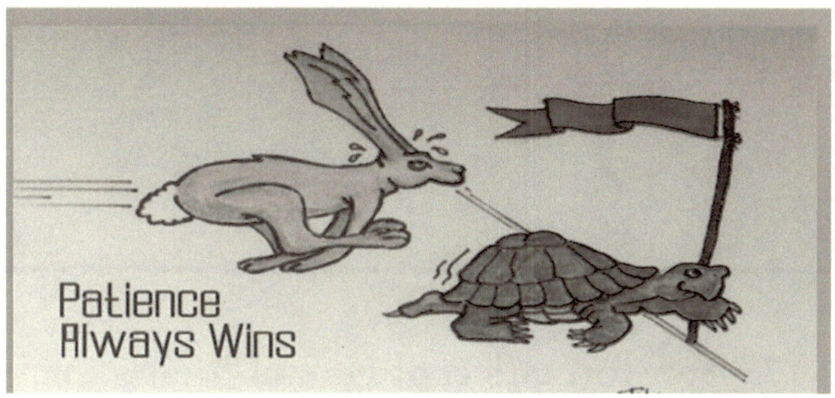

5. Installing Muscles is a Marathon Not a Sprint

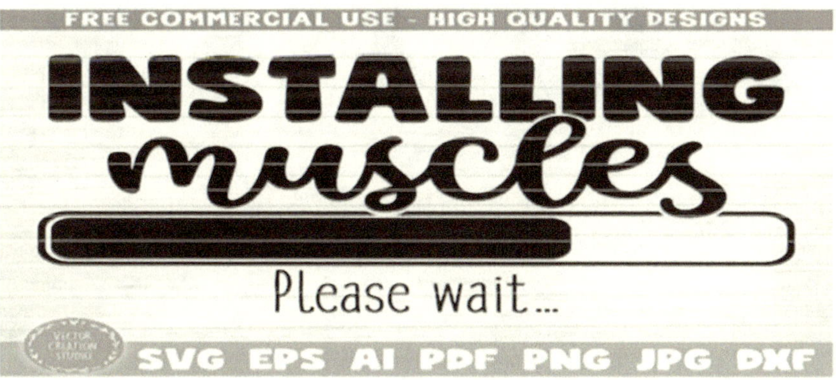

6. Only Facial Muscles Get Exercised

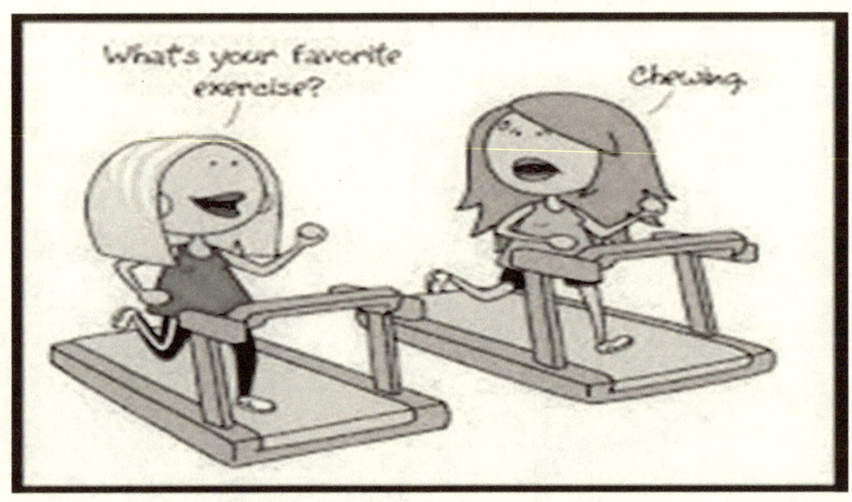

7. Transformation of Human Being-A Reality

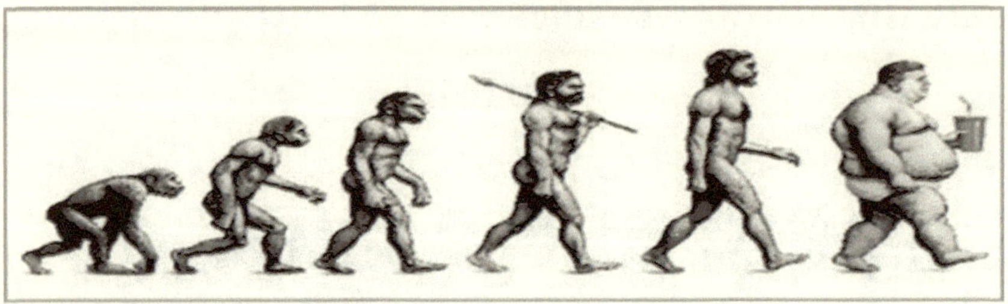

8. Imbalance Causes the Increase of Weight

YOUR FACE
when you realize your lunch would
take 200 burpees to burn off!

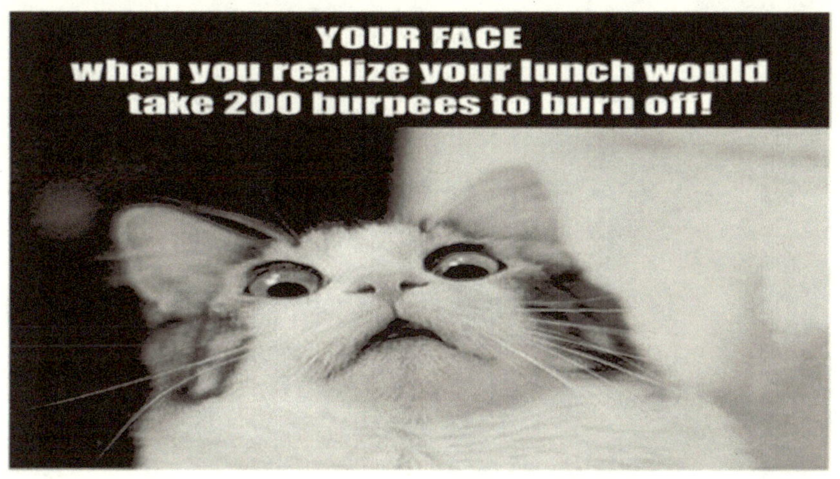

9. Need of the Hour-Control the Screen Time

THUMB OF THE RIGHT HAND GET MAXIMUM EXERCISE

The most beautiful parks in the middle of big cities

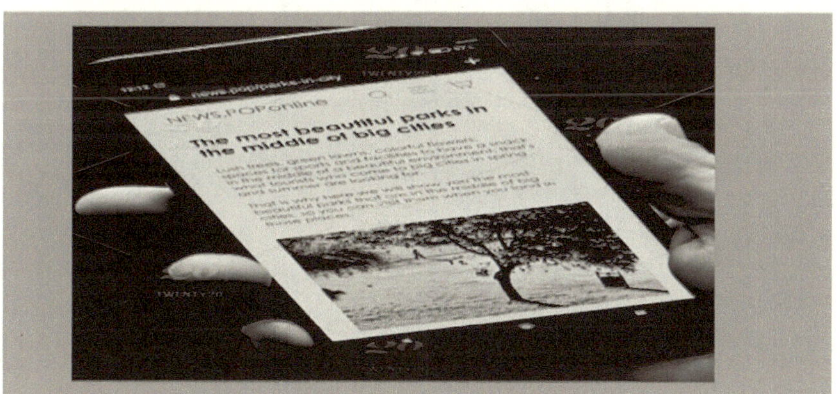

10. The Safest and Most Effective Method with Zero Side Effects

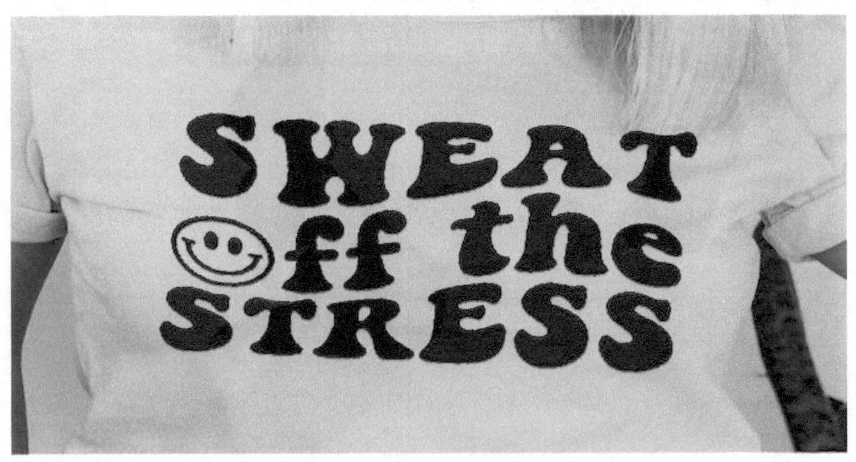

11. Walking Breaks are Necessary

SITTING CAN BE INJURIOUS

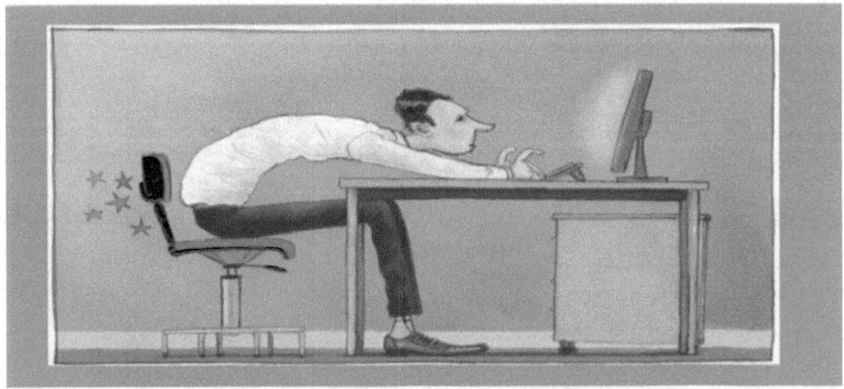

12. We Attack Heart By Lack of Execise and Improper Diet

HEART NEVER ATTACK

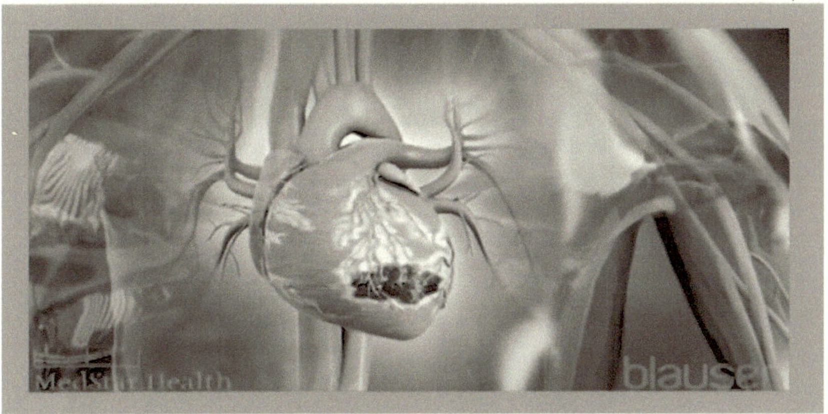

13. Drink Before Thirst

WATER IS INTERNAL AIR CONDITIONER

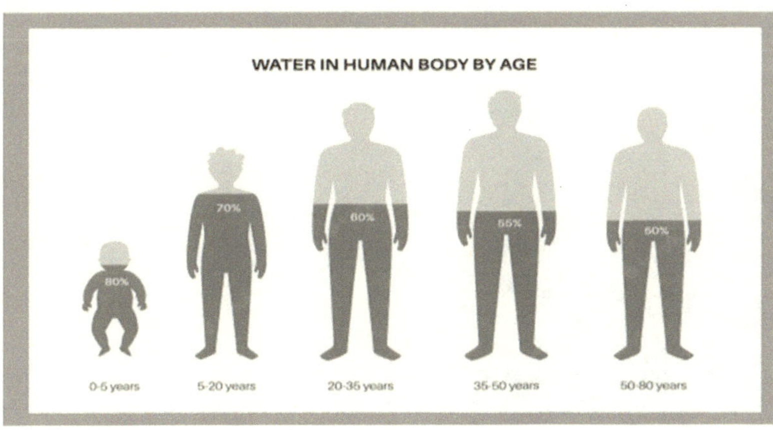

14. Pale Yellow Urine Indicates Proper Hydration

Drink More Water...

Your skin,
Your hair,
Your mind
and your body
will thank you

15. Consistent Effort Towards Fitness will Reap Rewards

YOU CAN SEE THE LIGHT AT THE LAST METER

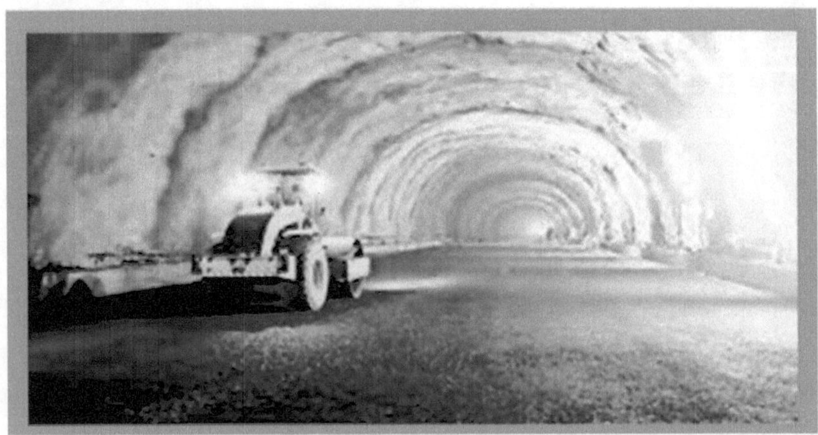

16. Embarking on a Fitness Journey is Ageless

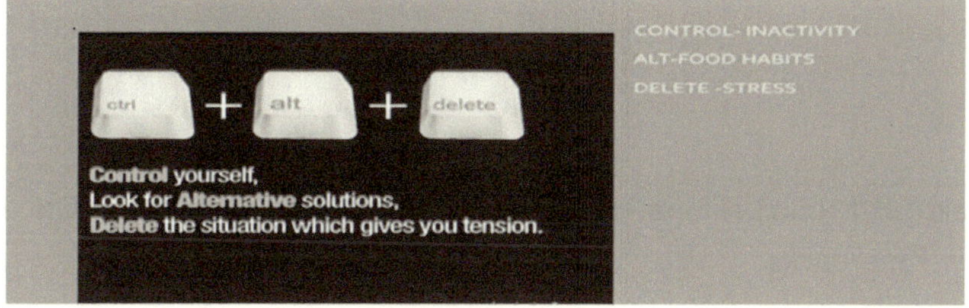

17. Don't Let Comparison Dampen Your Spirit; Remember, You are Blessed

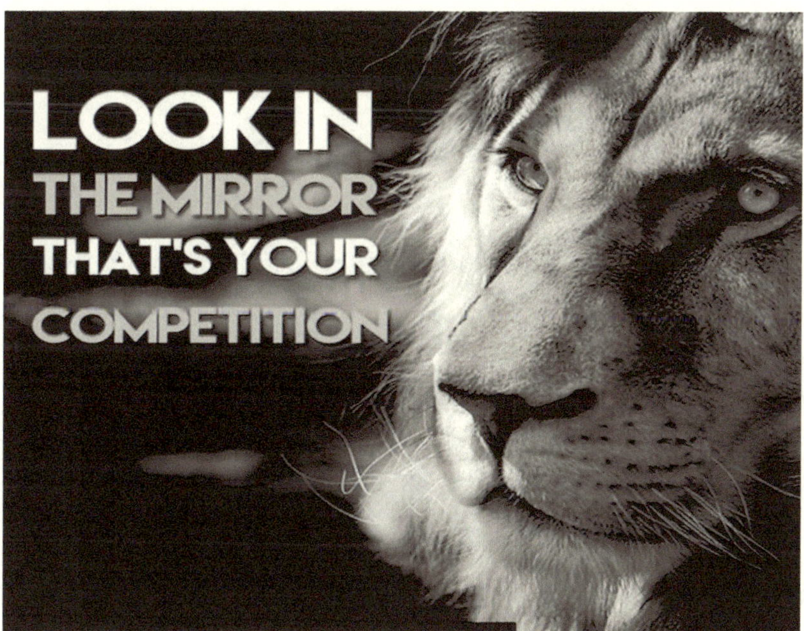

References

Bakru, H. K. (n.d.). Natural Home Remedies for Common Ailments. Orient Paperbacks.

Bhattacharya, A. (2017). Winning Like Virat: Think and Succeed like Kohli. Rupa Publications. ISBN-13: 978-8129146069

Crowley, C., & Lodge, H. S. (2007). Younger next year. Workman Pub Co. ISBN-13: 978-0761147732

Diamond, H., & Diamond, M. (2010). Fit for Life. Grand Central Life & Style. ISBN-13: 978-0446553643.

Diwekar, R. (2014). Do not lose out, work out. Westland. ISBN-13: 978-9383260959

Diwekar, R. (2018). Notes for Healthy Kids. Westland. ISBN-13: 978-938789452.

Diwekar, R. (2022). THE PCOD THYROID BOOK. Westland. ISBN-13: 978-9395073110.

Harchandrai, B. (2022). 5 Fingers of Fitness: A Fitness Love Story. ISBN-13: 978-8195088294.

Jain, N. (2015). 9To 5 Fit. Navbharat Sahitya Mandir. ISBN: 9789351980384.

Kshirsagar, D. S. G. (2015). The hot belly diet. Atria Books. ISBN-13: 978-1476734811

Mahawar, K. (2019). Fight With Fat: Battling India's Obesity Crisis. Fingerprint Publishing. ISBN-13: 978-9388810937.

Mathur, M. (2022). Honey it's not about six pack ABS. Notion Press.

Mogre, L. (2015). Total Fitness. Ebury Press. ISBN-13: 978-8184004366.

Mohapatra, B. M. S. (2019). Care for Your Health: A User Manual for Living Healthy. Notion Press.

Nambiar, S. (2018). Fit After 40: For a Healthier, Happier, Stronger You. Hachette India. ASIN: B07F8VKGL3.

Ojha, A., & Moitra, S. (2021). Fitness Habits-Breaking the barriers to fitness. Srishti Publishers & Distributors. ISBN-13: 978-9390441204

Otis, D. S. (2001). Staying fit after forty. Shaw Books. ISBN-13: 978-0877884538

Panday, D. (2013). Shut Up and Train! A Complete Fitness Guide for Men and Women. Random House India. ISBN-13: 978-8184003130

Patel, K. K. (2016). Athlete in You. Penguin Random House India. ISBN-13: 978-8184007091.

Purohit, N. (2021). The Lazy Girl's Guide to Being Fit. Penguin eBury Press. ISBN-13: 978-8184006018.

Rai, U. (2018). The fitness currency. Rupa Publications India. ISBN-13: 978-9353040758

Sah, S. K. (2013). Fitness simplified. Sterling Publishers. ISBN-13: 978-8120747814

https://chat.openai.com.

https://pubmed.ncbi.nlm.nih.gov/25559067/

www.brainyquotes.com

https://www.rd.com/article/workout-quotes/

https://parade.com/1045407/marynliles/fitness-quotes/

https://www.ncbi.nlm.nih.gov/pmc/articles/PMC3197470/

https://health.howstuffworks.com/wellness/diet-fitness/exercise-at-work/10-office-exercises-you-can-do-secretly.htm

https://steemit.com/physicalfitness/@tetas08/physical-fitness

https://www.shutterstock.com/image-vector/water-body-balance-by-age-h2o-2094429844

https://www.istockphoto.com/photos/digging-tunnel

www.ingramcontent.com/pod-product-compliance
Lightning Source LLC
LaVergne TN
LVHW091046150826
845673LV00002B/485

* 9 7 9 8 8 9 1 3 3 8 3 0 2 *